CAUGHT IN THE ACT

Forty Comic
Characters

For Readers
And Performers

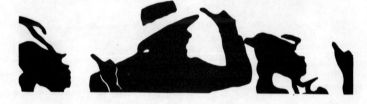

CAUGHT IN THE ACT

Forty Comic
Characters

For Readers
And Performers

by COREY REAY

Introduction by Charmion King

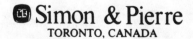 Simon & Pierre
TORONTO, CANADA

We would like to express our gratitude to The Canada Council and the Ontario Arts Council for their support.

Marian M. Wilson, Publisher

ISBN 0-88924-180-5
3 4 5 • 9 8

Canadian Cataloguing in Publication Data

Reay, Corey, 1961 –
Caught in the act : forty comic characters for readers and performers

ISBN 0-88924-180-5

I. Title.

PS8585.E19C38 1985   C812'.54   C85-099681-3   PR9199.3.R43C38 1985

General Editor: Marian M. Wilson
Editors: Roy Higgins and Sarah Robertson
Typesetting & Design: Cundari Group Ltd.
Printed and Bound in Canada

Simon & Pierre Publishing Co. Ltd.
P.O. Box 280 Adelaide St. Postal Stn.
Toronto, Ontario
Canada M5C 2J4

Only because of P.J. Lannon
can I say: this one's for Win Baine

Contents

Contents

Male

Acknowledgements

Some special thanks for support in many different ways ——
Barbara Baine and Bob Wenman — my mother and her favorite
  husband to date (mine too)
Glenn Wheeler — a saint despite himself
Kelly Mullaly and Martha Reilly — no them, no book
Duncan, John and Jane Spence — for friendship and canned goods
Denis Pizzacalla — also my mother
Charmion King — the first five letters say it all
Bryan Genesee — for his infectious ambition (I could use a dose)
The guinea pigs:
Jani Alison, Paul Amato, Ross Bryant, Kevin Bergsma, Deanne
Degruijter, Tracy Lynn Cochrane, Brock Johnston, Joanne McCarthy,
Daniel MacIvor, Carey Meltz, Kat Mullaly, Paul O'Sullivan, Shari
Robinson, Clifford Saunders, Robert Shipman, Steve Switzman,
Carol Thames, Jeff Wener, Michael Wile

Not to forget:
Shari and Marci Reay   Elsie Jeffreys
Joseph Shaw   Ernest J. Schwarz
Sally Edmunds   Reginald K. Dwight
David Gardner   Geoff Madison?
Francesca   Lenora Andruskevitch
Mark Redman   Arch McDonald
Tracy Woodrow   Niki Guadagni Benger
The Thompsi – Heidi, Megan and Shiona Sean Boyle
Laurie Thompson   J.C.
Dawn and Ted Eleco   Clyde Reay
Judy MacLaughlan   Roy Higgins
Dianne King (from a fan)   Sarah Robertson
Donny Quarles   Jean Paton
Dick and Ruth, the Reillys   and Marian Wilson

And all the rest: thank you

But most of all: Glen Williamson —— Where are you?

Introduction

by Charmion King

It is always a joy to come across a talent, and I have been fortunate to see some talented students while I have been teaching in the Theatre Department at George Brown College. All were performers. But a writer is a rare bird, and a comedic writer is practically an extinct species.

I had been teaching a course in Audition Technique at George Brown for several years, when, one day, a tall soft-spoken student, named Corey Reay, did a monologue for me that I did not recognize. Not only that, but it was marvelously funny. When I picked myself up off the floor and asked him what it was from, he told me he had written it himself. And that was the beginning of a very entertaining year for me.

Corey wrote monologues for everyone in that class. Some were lucky enough to have several written for them, and many of those pieces appear in this book. While they were written for specific people they do not require a rigid interpretation. I have seen a number of them, each performed by more than one person with very satisfying results — and each quite different. They are suitable for the young adult of the 80s who is no longer naive but who is still young.

A word of advice in preparing any of these pieces —— keep it light. There is a dark side to this humor. It is obvious when you read this book from beginning to end. The comedy lies in the desires and frustrations, not in the subtext of anger, fear and defeat.

Monologues from modern plays in the comedic or "light" vein are in short supply at the moment. Yet most artistic directors request a "classic" piece, a dramatic piece, and a "light" contemporary piece. So the aspiring actor is always presenting material that has no element of surprise, which, of course, is a major factor in comedy.

This collection offers some delightful alternatives.

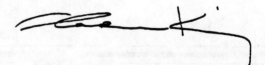

The Birth and Hard Times
of a Monologist

"I began as a union of an ovum and a sperm
and I've made little progress since.
I'm just a two legged slug with a penchant for ludes."

That's me quoting me — on me.
Welcome to my brain.
Come one, come all.
There's plenty of room.

In my second year of two at George Brown College, Toronto —
immersed in theatrical studies:
the pain ——
the joy ——
the endless orgies.
And, of course, the unrequested psychoanalysis —
always rendered axiomatically by middle-aged androgynies
who can't dress and haven't known a stable relationship
since the Mamas and Papas' last world tour.
Already up to my eyeballs in method and movement,
a fellow student added another challenge:
"Write me an audition monologue," she dared ——
And I did.

The monologue is back.
Great at parties, at the beach — or on the street passing a hat.
Put away the Twister —— let's mount a monologue.
What could be more uptown 80s than an entire theatrical
     production
from lights up to curtain down
that plays in less time than it takes to make toast?

You hold in your hand a year of my existence.
For the past twelve months I have lived and breathed monologues.
I have slept with them and eaten them.
Some read as if I'd passed them.
Those days after being at the same activity for longer than the
     average audition
I became distracted, irritable and fidgety
to the point of grand mal seizure.
It's not that writing them was a daily event.
Oh no.
Or a weekly ——
Or a monthly ——
Don't get me wrong.
That would require discipline.
Disci...what?
The actual time spent with a pen and paper was minimal ——
Which is my maximum.
It was the mental preoccupation that was oppressive.
These things were just always there.
A looming spectre ——
Something that had to get done.

The hardest part of writing,
like the hardest part of hairdressing —
is simply living.

As the year unfolds...
We meet me at school.
A fine place to be.
Safe and warm and satisfying —
like a uterus with a more attractive exit ——
Depending on how you look at it.
Nothing is asked of me — nothing do I give.
I am useless.
I am happy.
My paranoias are dormant — well, sluggish.
My neuroses bountiful but controlled.
My body saggy but clean.
I check my backyard for an apple tree with serpent ——
It's that good.

The monologues I write are calm and collected —
mirroring me ——
Parlor monologues.
The general note for them is:
In a smoking jacket with a café Viennese.
Voice insouciant — breathing easy.
Nudity when applicable ——
To my mind it always is.

Time?
It marches on and my college daze come to an end.

The plug is pulled.
Paradise is lost — again.
I'm out of school and on the streets.
Cars are everywhere — horns beeping — drivers yelling ——
I've joined the human race.
It's cold and harsh and you quite often have to use
unattractive exits to get places ——
Depending on how you look at it.
There I was:
No job.
No future.
Just a statistic — a number.
I was a four.
The general note for the monologues at this point in the journey is:
"Aaaaaaaa."
My head's a mess, my nerves an overloaded jumble ——
Alcohol seems in order.

Yes indeed:
I did the town.
The town did me.
I brought to fruition my infantile fantasies
of one day waking in strange places
with unfamiliar faces
in apartments owned by pimps ——
Dreams really do come true.
I'm remembering that moment as a boy — oh, 6 or 7 —
gleefully skipping along — passing the men on Sally Ann's steps ——
"Someday," my sweet voice sang, "I'm going to be just like you."

Where happy little blue birds fly...

Yes indeed:
It's summertime in the big town and the monologues are mean ——
The spewage of a sautéed brain.
For two months I find nothing funny but incontinence in the face
    of adversity
and non-committal fornication between consenting adults.
To the average 13-year-old boy, I was a comic genius.

Monologues?
No monologues.
I just went to bed and watched the leaves blow by.
That was the fall.
And then? ——
I got up.
And the world said, "Season's greetings."
I just gave it a dirty look.

Christmas time: the joy of getting.
Christmas time: the joy of family.
14 cousins — all under 10 — sense my lack of interest
and I'm buried in a mountain of vengeful yuppie droppings.
For this the Lord has come?
Christmas time: the dressing is wonderful
and I'm an angry young man — in a full grown snit ——
Poor dear.
Why?
Because it's not turning out the way I'd planned.
I'm over 21 and I still have to work.
No Jag.
Every minute problem I see as colossal.
Nothing is minor, except a few casual aquaintances.
Poor and powerless...

A lintball on a sweater
takes on the gravity of a job lost
due to terminal illness.
My mind wanders to a day of peace in the world —
a Jag in the driveway and tickets to Rio in the armoire ——
Lintballs would be lintballs
and terminal illness just one of those things.
Poor me.
One wreck on a planet full of them —
with nowhere to turn for pity
without having to return the favor.
"You and me both, pal, you and me both."

Finally?
A small inner voice said, "We are your brain cells — we are few.
Cheer up — nothing could be this bad" ——
And it couldn't.
The monologues are coming and the note says:
Do them in the parlor
with a beer in one hand and an Earl Grey in the other.

We've come full circle.
So had I.
A synthesis of who I once was and what I'd been through since.
Like me — like my monologues.
And somewhere in there a nice lady gave me some money
and said she'd publish this book.
May she die wealthy at 200 having lost her figure at 194.
I thought you should know.
Somehow it's all in here.

One remarkable thing worth noting, by way of a significant PS,
is that most of this action took place in my head ——
Where most bad things do.
The rest of the world missed the fun — too busy having its own.
Through most of it, humanity saw me as it always has and will ——
Some liking — some loving ——
Most indifferent.
You and me both.

That is the struggle that runs throughout this work:
The never ending battle between who others think we are —
and who we believe we really are.
And more:
Who we think we are and who we really are.
What seems and what is.
Laws deal in "is" — discos in "seems."
Pop tarts having nothing to do with either of them ——
God love 'em.
At this point in my life, that struggle holds my attention like
    nothing else can —
except the Flintstones.
Yes indeed:
Since the first amoeba split in two
and pondered the cruel inequity of asexual reproduction ——
Life's been a bitch.
The best we can do is say: "so be it" — and laugh.
All the people in this book know that.

Love me — love my monologues.
Enough said.

Foreword

Make of these pieces what you will.
What you can ——
You bought 'em.
I give very few notes because you'd probably ignore them anyway.
Intelligent actors will always make their own decisions.
That's the way it should be.
That's what makes theatre worth watching.
I'm not — however — above hinting.
So:
I think most of these should be played straight.
The way I hear them — monkeys could do them.
Monkeys have.
I say just play them.
Simply do 'em.

However:
You may not hear them the way I do and you may want to
     characterize them.
Fine by me.
Do them in full Cossack regalia with a Teutonic lilt
if you think it's best for you.
Make adjustments, even repairs, if you think a piece needs them —
always keeping in mind rhythm and tone.
If I've written a line that is nothing short of traumatic for you
     to play ——
Cut it.

I'll never know.
My spy network is a very small affair.
Many young actors have a strange belief that to change an
author's words
is a grave artistic immorality.
Most authors believe this too.
But:
Short of totally misrepresenting an author's ideas, that's not so.
What I'm on about here are those finicky little things in a
    speech or line
that an actor wishes beyond all measure could be changed ——
I say change 'em.
You'll have enough to worry about.
Are they laughing at me?
Do they think I have no talent?
That I am a gross parody of what an actor really is? ——
Things like that.

Another hint:
A joke is not a mountain to be scaled.
A sonorous crescendo.
It shouldn't build like a rocket launch.
Like an orgasm.
No joke is as good as an orgasm — although I'm just a man.
A joke should come and go.
A painless needle prick administered by the hand of a firm,
    confident, ugly nurse.
Over in flash.
Don't march through a joke with a huge half-time band singing:
"Here comes a funny one — boy are you going to laugh, do wat
    diddy."

Because they may not laugh.
They may not even smirk ——
They may shout "next."
Sail through a joke.
Just say it — don't mount it.
Don't tell an audience that something is funny — they'll decide
    for themselves.
And remember:
There is no universal sense of humour and no universally funny
joke.
Be prepared for that.
Let it comfort you.
Let it make you not ask for your money back.

Finally:
I'm a Canadian.
Head to toe — all parts in between...
From St. Catharines, Ontario: the Garden City —
now domiciled in Toronto: the Good City.
So:
I use local images and locales
that may mean Detective Tracy's first name to you.
There aren't many, but those there are — feel free to change them.
Make them suit the occasion.
For example:
When I say Kenora, Ontario, if I were American I would mean
    Tonawanda, New York —
and when I say Al Waxman what I really mean is Anson Williams.
    Etc....

And so —
I wish you luck ——
You're on your own.

Somewhere in time...
Somewhere in Toronto
where I live
in relative obscurity —
in absolute poverty...
For nibbling at both —— thanks.

Corey Reay

FEMALE

1

Ivory Girl

Hunny, hunny, hunny.
It's all very simple.
This is a bottle of gin.
That is tonic.

I have mixed both together in this glass.
I have put in this green thing which is lime.
And all of them together...in one big beautiful motion
I have passed over my lips, over my gums.
Look out stomach ——
Here it comes.

It's called drinking.
And this is the one after my third.
Care to tell me how many the next will make?
It's not that much.
If I were a man you wouldn't think twice about it.

Ah, but I'm not — am I?
I'm a woman — aren't I?
What's worse — I'm a white woman.
I'm the color of lilies and I have two pert breasts.
Lucky me ——
Lucky you.

I'm just so pretty.
Let's face it — I'm gorgeous.
I'm a piece.
I am still young — and I am a piece.
Wanna squeeze?
Of course you don't; the sun's still out ——
That would be dirty.

Hey, that's it — isn't it?
You're upset because there's nothing uglier in the entire universe
Than a drunk white woman
Alone on a Tuesday afternoon.
Is there.
It is grotesque, isn't it?
I just may be sick.
How about you?

What's wrong with me?
This little WASP bitch should be doing the laundry.
I should be in a tizzy — an absolute quandary.
I missed the rinse cycle for the fabric softener.
Oh no ——
She shrieks.
Now I'll have to use the dryer sheets.
Oh no.
Now she's done it.
She doesn't have any dryer sheets.
All the clothes will be rock hard.
Static cling everywhere.
Underwear hanging onto towels and socks fused onto pants.
Think of the mayhem.

Poor little Jenny will be off to school with her little skirt
Sticking to her scabby little legs.
She'll be the butt of cling jokes.
Poor thing ——

The little shit.
Let her clean her own clothes.

That's what's really wrong, isn't it?
I'm not playing my part.
I should be preparing a fondue.
I should be refilling the soft soap container in the guest bathroom.
It's awfully low you know.

Yes, the possibilities are endless.
Why as we speak I could be cataloguing coupons ——
What fun.
Constantly new vistas opening.
It's just too much.
And yet — you know — here I am.
With my gin and tonic and my fantasies.
Today it was John Paul II.
It was a religious experience let me tell you.
He's quite a Pole.
He's gentle — but firm.
And flattering ——
He told me I was the best in 47 different languages.

I'm going to burn, aren't I?

You see hunny, hunny, bunny, booby wooby ——
It's not enough.
This lovely house.
The big hole in the backyard filled with water ——
It's not enough.
If you're married to plankton, then maybe ——
But you're not.
I'm more than that.
Much more.
And I'm never more than that
Than after a trip to the liquor cabinet
On a weekday afternoon.

Welcome home, hunny.
Did you have a nice day?

You Can't Take It With You

I'm sitting here.
Pacing here.
Flailing here — little pieces of me dying with each passing second —
and you're somewhere waiting for a bus?
My sanity hinges on public transit?
I don't believe you sometimes, Trish.
What does friendship mean to you? I'll tell you what it means
     to me ——
I'm sorry — I'm ranting — I'm sorry.
Just sit down, OK?
Please sit down ——
Bend at the knee.
Thanks.

Alright —— Oh God, I feel like such trash, Trish.
White trash.
I never knew what that was before — but now I do.
I found out the hard way.
Don't say a thing.
Don't say, "What happened?" and "Oh my God," like that.
Alright — Alright — alright —— Shut up.
I'll tell.
OK — here it is and it's not very nice.
Trish, you're gonna hate me.
It's gonna fill you with disgust.

Years from now, people will mention my name
   and you'll spit —— oooh, sorry — gross.

I want you to know that you've been a good friend.

Alright, I'll get to the point.
I went out on a date.
There's more, you idiot.
I went out on a date — but who with?
Don't guess, this isn't Trivial Pursuit, Trish.
This is reality.
I went out on a date with...Gary the Giver.

I knew I could depend on you for such a mature reaction, Trish.
Take your finger out of your mouth.
I know he's gross.
I know he's an unthinkable.
Anyway, Trish — there's more.
I said don't say, "Oh my God" — 'cause you don't even know
   what it is ——
Even though you probably do.

Trish...it's gone Trish.
It's lost forever.
I did it with a person called Giver.
I'm gotten, Trish.
I'm spent — used.
Label me slut.
Oh yuk.
What a slime he is.
What a slime I am.

Ah Trish, I lost it in the back of a Ranchero
with a man who has "Eat Me" tattooed on his arm.
A guy who owns one pair of socks.

Maybe I'm a nympho.
There was no love.
No love.
Nothing — special.
No candles — no wine — no fireplace — no Duran Duran.
I don't know how I could do it.
He just said all the right things.
He's good with words and there's something there that the eye
    just can't see —
and it just — I didn't think — and ——
I don't know.

Trish, the point is that I was deflowered by a Neanderthal
    with my free will urging me on.
I am a nympho — like my cousin Trudy, Trish.
I'm trash.
The only good thing is that I hated every second of it.
I'll never do it again —— it's horrible.
Trish, my innocence is gone — and I want it back.

What do you mean?
Of course I'm still going to the concert tonight.
Jeez.

The Sellout

Do you ever think there's something "deficit" in what we do?
Something wrong, even dangerous?

I'll have a margarita please.

Two please.
What a rear view.

I got into advertising because I couldn't make a living as a
    playwright.
In fact — I couldn't make a thing.
And — I like to make a living because it feeds me; and it pays
for my Lamborghini, my sojourns on the Riviera ——
and I love being able to say:
"My cleaning girl is coming in on Thursday."

But I did start with values.
Good ones.
I wanted to say a lot and I had a lot to say, and that never
    included —
"Static Gone: It takes the sting out of static cling."
Do you know how much money I made on that one?
Botswana has a smaller national budget.
It's not fair.
It's crazy.

I have friends who write entire novels and make not one-tenth
of what I do for 30 seconds of dialogue.
But they have something I don't ——
Respect.
Of other people and for themselves.
And we don't have it because — let's face it ——
We don't deserve it.
What we do is silly.
I don't know if I can live with that anymore.
Yes I can.

Thank you.
Run a tab please.

What a god.

There was a time in my rebellious adolescence when I courted
    communism.
Oh gasp. Pinko me.
And now I'm a full-time instrument of the capitalist system.
A betrayal of my youth.
That's not good for one's mental health.
I helped create the most effective way
of influencing and warping the human mind ever devised:
The TV commercial.
Sensory deprivation with great production values.
When people ask me what I do for a living, sometimes I just say:
"I insult intelligence."

Just once I'd like to do an honest, realistic commercial.
For toilet paper, let's say.
"This is toilet paper and its purpose is to clean shit off your bum.
And you should use ours because we get it the cleanest
in the fewest wipes."

There'd be line-ups around the block for the stuff.
Let the competition convince them to buy it because it feels nice.
Which is so ridiculous.
People don't take the Pepsi Challenge by dipping their fingers in it.
You don't judge a new car by smelling it.
People don't —— They know.
They know what makes one tampon or sanitary napkin
superior to the competition isn't a floral package
or how well some blonde big-breasted,
far-too-pretty for her own good, teenage girl
        can roller-skate while she uses them.

Just once —— oh, I'd love to do this.
Insert the name of a tampon in the place of an oven cleaner
and send them the copy ——
"Look — after two hours: first their brand, now ours."

Come on — I'm as much of a lady as the next guy
and I know my sensibilities could take it
if someone pointed out on TV
the often overlooked fact that the purpose of lady's napkins
        is absorbency.
Look, if Bounty can do it —
Let's see Kotex take the teacup test.

Oh, look, I've got to get back.
It's rent week.
The best excuse I know
for living with no respect and exploiting the masses.

The Immaculate Misconception

It's all image.
I don't know where it came from, I've just always had it.
And I hate it.
The whole world thinks I'm something I'm not:
Clean, pure, willingly chaste.
Morality hangs over me like a cloud.
I make people nervous.
My own parents whisper around me.
As a child nobody wanted to play with me; they wanted to pray
    to me.
I make everyone feel guilty.
Pregnant women turn away from me in shame.
Prostitutes throw themselves over puddles for me to walk on.
I've never seen my own dog lick himself —— he goes into the
    next room.
Oh, I get so mad sometimes, and I want to swear — but I can't.
I did once and everyone who heard was found dead within a week.
Valium, natural gas and a running car in a closed garage,
    respectively.

I'm the immaculate misconception.
My own rabbi told me to become a nun.
I'll never be able to make love.
The only person who came close — couldn't.
You could see it in his eyes ——

It was like asking him to rape Mother Theresa.
So close, so very close.

It's not fair.
I never asked for this.
It's not fair.
There are so many things I want to do, so many places I want to
    go ——
But who's going to take the Virgin Mary mud wrestling?
You know, every time I hear a brass instrument, I break out in a
    cold sweat.
It's the Angel Gabriel, I think, and he's come with a little
    proposition.
It's the Holy Ghost, and he's come to get it on ——
"Oh no," I think.
"Not me. You've got the wrong person."

Inside here is a lascivious pig, longing for freedom —
wanting to run naked through the streets,
scaring little children and kicking old women,
and losing my virginity again and again and again.
Going into head shops and buying pipe screens and lollipops
    shaped like genitalia, and entering wet T-shirt contests
and shaking them and shaking them,
with crowds of randy young men screaming: "Yes! Go! Yes! Yes!"

We all have our dreams.
Our little fantasies.
Just don't bet your ass that they're going to happen ——
Pardon me.

It's a Living

Talk?
Well, OK — for a minute.
OK, shoot.

Why do I do what I do?
Hmm. Well, I wish I could give you a sad story
about a mixed up childhood or poor self-respect —
You know, being raped and liking it,
or a total lack of belief in my ability to do anything else.
But — I can't.
That's just not the way it is.
I mean, I did come from a broken family, but who doesn't anymore?
Its value for getting people to feel sorry for you
is next to worthless.

It just so happens that late in my teens
I decided I wanted to go to college — and I had no money and, well,
everything I'd need was right there and there. *(Indicates her breasts)*
So, I got into the business.
And I made the money to go to school.
It's a movie of the week.

You a writer?
Oh.
Well, I became a nurse. I am a nurse.

The joke on the street is:
"Not only can she give you a dose, but she can cure it too."
And it is — only a joke.
Yes, I'm also known as Florence Who Nightly Wails.
I don't mind. I like it.
Well, anyway, there I was, having to watch people shit,
giving them sponge baths and enemas — and I thought:
"Hell, I could be doing this very same thing and making eight
    times the money."
I like helping people but I wasn't helping myself very much.
But doing this is helping people.
Making life a little easier for an hour.
Taking a load off the consciences of the frigid housewives of the
    world.
All quite noble.
So, I got out of the hospital and back on the street.
And I like it.
I'm good at it ——
I am.

It's interesting too, you know, how you get to see the other side
    of people ——
The side you don't see at work or in stores or in restaurants.
Everyone being totally civilized.
Then there's the other side ——
The one that comes out when they're completely naked
with someone who will do sexually anything they want —
    almost anything.
That's when people are really fascinating.
'Cause that's when they're really themselves.
No bullshit.
You know?

So enough of me talking.
Are we going somewhere?
Hey, hey — let's see what time it is ——
Oh looky, it's 11:00 — and it's Tuesday.
You are in luck.
Tuesday from 11:00 till Wednesday at 6:00 I have a half-off sale.
Lucky, lucky you.

Hey, where you going?
What's wrong?
Not good enough for you?
Maybe you couldn't get it up if we did!
Who wants your little stinky dinky anyway?
Get out of here.

Pig!

Oh, hi.
How are you?
Want some company?

Infighting

Oh, there they go.
It's not serious.
Just embarrassing.
I'm sorry.
Just another playing of the Randall family's modern adaptation of
    The Taming of the Shrew.
It's a family tradition.
No, habit actually.
Addiction really.
It's the same fight every time.
Same attacks.
Same defenses.
My mother will get it all out of her system and then start
    brooding about it again tomorrow.
The subject is my father's mistress.
Oh, don't pretend; I know you know ——
Everyone does.
My father has a squeeze on the side.
It's common knowledge.
Check public washrooms for references.

Well, my mother for some reason known only to her chooses to
    stay with him.
I would have given him 60 seconds to pack, leave the charge
    cards and hit the road.

But not my mom.

Did you hear that?
Where do they learn language like that?

Anyway, as for my dad,
well sometimes I can't blame him for keeping Melanie.
That's his bimbo.
Melanie Dunkirk.
She's beautiful.
She really is.
If I ever become a lesbian, I'll want her too.
I've met her lots of times.
Not what you'd call an engaging conversationalist.
But my father says, "That's not her purpose."
Sometimes I think my dad forgets after all is said and done —
I am a woman too.
And I wish that when he gets the urge to say things like that,
    he'd control himself.

Oh, but I do see his side.
My mother used to be beautiful.
But she — she — she's not anymore.
I think it started when she was carrying me.
She got so used to eating for two that she just couldn't give it up.
Sometimes I think she just doesn't realize what a buffalo she's
    become.
I think it would do her a lot of good if someone very bluntly said —
"Betty, look, you have the figure of a snowman."
But it's not going to be me.
I have too much to lose.

Ah — quiet.
It means one of two things: one of them is lying dead out there
or my father has just promised to buy my mother a new fur.
Nothing can shut my mother up quite like the skin of a dead
    animal.
My father's body is so hairy
    that I once suggested when he dies
    she could make a coat out of him.
Neither of them found it very funny.

Now —— if you'll excuse me for a minute.
I have to go in there.
It's time for my part in the play.
It's the teen-troubled-by-her-parents-arguing scene.
It's good for a couple of bucks.

After all — I am my mother's daughter.

The Manic

Do you realize what that means?
I can't be happy unless I'm depressed.
How's that for neurotic?
It means, that either consciously or unconsciously I have to spend
    my entire life —
in search of disaster.
Pain is my pastime.
Although, sometimes I look around and I think it's not just me.
It's everyone.
Why else would we live in a world of smoking, marriage, pregnancy,
and Dino De Laurentis films?
I think we all need to suffer.
Without it we're bores.
No wonder North Americans can be such tedious company.
Our good fortune denies us the very basic horrors nature intends
    for us:
Starvation, exposure, hand-washing dishes ——

Which reminds me. Get some Cascade.

I mean, how can people be expected to have a personality
with Daddy's Visa card in their pockets? ——

Would you please remind me to tell my father about the coat?
Thanks.

My favorite method of self-destruction is probably the oldest and
        most common ——
Falling in love.
That great intangible that makes well-adjusted human beings
endow others of the species, often of a lesser quality —
with the ability to walk on water.

It's such a strange paradox.
The only thing more harrowing than being in love is not being
        in love.
It offers more opportunities for self-pity, feelings of inadequacy,
        rejection, anger and plain old depression
than anything else the human condition can produce
— including family reunions.
I highly recommend it.
The ensuing pain of unrequited love is to be thanked for some
        of the best literature, art, music
and dinner conservation ever produced ——

More potatoes, veal?

I have consistently assured myself of love's maximum pain potential
by always falling for people certain not to fall for me.
People of whom even my mother says, "You haven't got a chance."
And since most relationships are built on a foundation of
        physical attraction —
I always direct my affections towards people
who are far better looking than me.
People who I know would giggle at the sight of my unclothed body.
People who have already giggled at the sight of my clothed body.
But the most accommodatingly tragic group to fall for
are people we are already friends with.

You know the conversation:
"Lately I've been feeling differently about our relationship."
"Oh?"
"Yes...I - I - I"
"Oh!"
"I - I - I - I'm in love with you...how do you feel?"
"Oh, of course I love you too."
"Oh!"
"Yes — like a sister."
"Bastard."

I have an extended family that could fill a football stadium ——

John?
John?
Are you sure you won't have any more?

John — I think there's a way you could help me be a very
    interesting person.
Oh, I haven't even asked the question but I already know your
    answer.
And I'm already feeling upset.
I'm feeling it already.
I'm feeling the need to write a poem about this.
It's a horrible feeling because I write horrible poetry.
You don't want to be the cause of more bad poetry do you?
There's enough in this world already by all gay men over 20 and
    all straight females under it...

Oh no.
You can't.
Don't say yes.

I'll be so happy.
I'll become the most boring, civilized person the world's ever known.
I'll go to bed at nine.
Make my bed.
Go to the zoo.
I'll stop neglecting my grandmother.
I'll wanna talk about the most boring, inane things all the time
    — like the weather, actors.
I'll start conversations with complete strangers — in bank queues
    — at bus stops —
Places where only the mentally ill ever initiate conversation.
I'll eat nothing but finger sandwiches.

Oh no, please just say you're not sure.
Let's keep me fascinating.

Man's Best Friend

Wait.
Wait.
Stop.
You're making it difficult.
Please.

Thank you. I think I made a mistake.
Look, before we take this any further — I have to warn you
about the risk you're about to take with your...manhood.
It's on the block ——

Now, I know that as we speak,
you are probably the most heterosexual mammal to grace this couch
since my Uncle Harry, Fart King of Forest Hill, last Christmas.
The abused Leafs T-shirt, the mismatched cords, the Brut,
Springsteen as a background to foreplay —— it's all there.
You are M-A-N and God bless you for it.
Your body is almost literally nothing but testosterone.
Wherever your sweat touches me — hair begins to grow.
But, what you have here — in your arms and in your mouth ——
Is a woman with a talent.
Thank you, thank you, that's very nice...
But I mean a different sort of talent.
Curse is a better word for it.
No, no — that's worse. This isn't a trip down Judaic law.
Curse is the wrong word.

Let's go back to talent.
No...gift. Gift is good.
I am a woman with a gift and you are a man with a problem ——
That is — not you — but what I may do to you.
I'm exciting myself —— it's not coming out right.
It's just that I seem to have the touch that kills.
That kills; that's it.
That kills that thing called desire
that all sorts of men have for women.
The touch that changes —— that's better.
That changes men who like women into men who like men...a lot.
Too much for TV.
Oh, I know what you're thinking: not me — I'm a man — all
    man ——
But that's what they all thought.
Yes, all of them.
Gone over to the other side.
Ran over with a look on their face as if they'd smelled
    something bad.
They had —— *moi*.
Sally the Sea Creature.
Henrietta Highliner.
Their last ugly brush with bush.

We just start to make love and a little light goes off — it's there
    in their eyes ——
a little voice pipes up inside and they're thinking,
"What the hell am I doing with this thing? I'm going to Ralph's.
These hips are unreasonable —— she's got no dink — balls, yes..."
Oh, I don't know what I do —— it's so depressing.
I tell a man I'm attracted to him and within seconds,
for the first time in his life — he's assessing fabric textures

and trying to decide what color to do the breakfast nook in.
A breakfast nook he doesn't even have yet.
Giorgio Armani owes me more than he'll ever know.

My last boyfriend: a pig.
A baseball freak —— hairy and loud — horribly insensitive —
     with smelly feet ——
A dreamboat.
The best sex since the Gauls sacked Rome.
The man was merciless. I had to keep cat gut on the bed table.
He was wonderful.
Two weeks, two weeks, that's all it took — of intensive me.
He traded in his suits for blue jeans, Levi shirts and Nikes
with the tongues up — shaved his chest — cut his hair   —
     quit his firm —
works as a waiter and weeps heavily at anything with subtitles ——
And he thanks me.
He's not welcome.

Look — I'm not nuts.
I'm just observing a very real pattern and I felt you should know
     about it.
It's only fair.
With that said — I'm all yours ——
Be mean.

Pardon?

Yes, this is *L'Air du Temps* I'm wearing.
I'll get your coat —— No, better yet...
I'll go get us some spritzers
while you rearrange the furniture and house plants.
Won't that be fabulous?

The Winner

I've worked hard all my life.
Everything I had I earned.
More tea?
It's that Earl Grey.
I don't like it myself — but it's all part of my new image.
So's your magazine.
I'd never heard of it till the other day.
The man who decorated the new house said I should get some
    for the coffee table.
I said I'd never read them and he said he was quite certain of that —
but that's not what they're there for.
Well your's was one he recommended, and it looks very pretty
    there — doesn't it?

Thanks.

I guess you want to know about the changes.
There have been so many.
People who say winning a lottery won't change them into
    different people
have either never won or they're full of shit.
The second I found out I turned into a completely different person.
A much better person than I used to be —
and a much better person than anyone I used to know.
And all the unselfish things that people say they'll do with the money...
Forget it, honey.
I won it and it's mine.

You may have noticed that my children aren't here.
I told you on the phone I have three.
Let me tell you about my kids.
They're rotten.
Their teacher used to call me all the time to tell me how rotten
    they were.
As if I didn't know.
Once the principal from their school called to get permission to
    give the oldest the strap.
Well, I said, "Of course" — but could he wait so I could come
    down and cheer?
It's not completely their fault.
Their fathers were pigs.
Anyway — as soon as the cheque was cashed
they were packed off to a private boarding school hours from here.
Yes, there are so many advantages to having money.
So many things I want to do with it.
So many people I'd love to hurt.
You see, I figured out that the only type of legal revenge
that average people like you and me can get on other people
...is economic.
You can't hit them.
I couldn't knock them off. I was raised a Christian.
But with enough money you can deprive them of their livelihoods.
And that you can do by buying the restaurant
where you slaved your ass off for 8 long years
and going up to the filthy, grabbing, miserable puke who was
    your boss
and canning him on the spot.
My dear, money is marvelous.

How about a beer.
I have Heineken.

Family Planning

Frank.
I think our problem here is the different conception we each have
of what constitutes a satisfied woman.
Mine —— rooted in mid 1985.
Yours —— in late 1643.
To you I can't possibly be a whole, complete, satisfied person
until I bear a baby — can I?
I have to breed, reproduce, carry on the species —
especially that part of the species with your last name —
before that can happen.
Correct? ——

Well —— no go, Frank.
Here I stand, a finished product — *sans bambino*,
and very enthusiastically on the pill.
Which I have no intention of going off.
Because this is my body and I decide what and who gets inside of it.
And most importantly: who lives inside of it.
So my life is going to continue as is — selfishly.
I'm going to continue building status, position, making bucks —
being, in short, a very successful man — until I — not us —
    decide that it's time
to become a successful penisless person as well.

So — pack up your arguments, Frank, because I'm not going to budge.
You can go on and on about your mother this, and your mother
     that —
about what children brought her ——
How she grew stronger and more hearty after each successive baby.
How pregnancy made her glow and shine.
Because while I know it's the story of true womanhood to you ——
It's actually the story of a radioactive rabbit on steroids.
And Frank — we can also forget about how she gave birth to
     your brother — all by herself —
and about her two caesarians — which I'm sure she also did by
     herself —
because Frank —— I'm not your mother.
I'm not hearty the way your mother is.
Horses are — a good chili can be.
But this babe ain't.

Which leads me to another consideration.
It may sound narcissistic, but in addition to the sacrifice
     of career and social life,
there's also the end of my body as we know it to consider.
This fine figure of mine that I have spent an entire lifetime
     to create and maintain.
This marvelous shape that I have denied myself billions
     of calories for, jogged millions of miles for,
          received untold numbers of leering, disgusting comments for ——
I will not jeopardize.
I am not about to waste a lifetime of yogurts and aerobics —
     and I hate them both —
by allowing a human being to take up residence inside me
and turn the smooth tight skin of my torso
into a reasonable facsimile of a road map of Regina.
I won't do it ——

And don't forget, Frank — though as a man I'm sure you have —
that even after I have endured those long nine months
as a bloated invalidic life support system ——
The little bugger still has to get out.
And that is one exit that is going to cause me one hell of a lot
    of pain.
Pain notwithstanding — there's also the damage to consider.
You see, since my little exit route
has so far been exclusively a one-way street
with — and let's be honest here — relatively light traffic...
When that darling eight pound parasite decides it's time
to make the break and smell the roses —
its little head is going to turn my small one-way street
into a major four-lane highway.
I have no intention of spending the prime of my life
with my genitalia dangling to my knees.
Which is, of course, an exaggeration — which is to say —
I just can't do it...now.
I love children.
I'm not a witch.
Maybe some day I'll want one of my own — just not yet.

Alright Frank — stop moping.
Lift up your head.
Let's go to bed.

Mother Knows Best

I don't want to lecture you.
I went through a similar phase.
I understand.
We were raised in a land where you couldn't have sex in all the
    ways you wanted
until you were 21 — and even then — the other person had to
    consent to it.

So — when our time came — some of us took just a little
    advantage of our new right.
We considered it a license to abandon our usual concepts of
    morality and behaviour —
society's image of what was decent and religion's of what was
    sinful —
in favor of doing it with everyone we possibly could.

Now, now dear. I know it sounds harsh when put so bluntly,
but again — I'm not lecturing you.
Only trying to relate.

There was a time when I was by day a serious, efficient, career
    women of the 80s
and by night a rabid hedonistic bar wench.
Which is not to say that that is what you've become.
You're certainly on your way but this isn't a judgement call.

I couldn't do that without being a hypocrite.
In those days I had sex in great quantities.
Let's not talk numbers.
It was just so easy.
The men were there — I was there.
What else was there to do?
The conversation was dull — too scripted.
Besides — the more they'd say, the less attractive they'd seem to
    become.
A man you approached because of his brawny, masculine
    appearance
turned out to be more feminine than you were.
Or the sensitive, tweed-clad intellectual
you sent knowing glances to over your tipped glass all evening
turned out to be an inane sadist
whose break-the-ice line was, "Want to be spanked bitch?"
Well, I rarely did.

Why, dear, why do we do it?
I suppose some of us enjoy waking up in the morning feeling
    cold and empty,
but feeling a warm body beside us when we do.
And some of us, burdened with great depth and sensitivity —
    and I include you —
simply like to rebel now and then and act as shallow as we can.
Our little way of saying "Up yours" to civilization.
So you see — I've been there.
Even now — yes, when your father's going through one of his
    little dry spells —
which can sometimes last months — I find myself thinking of the
    old days: the evil 80s — looking at men intently, constantly
    — undressing them with my eyes, visually caressing their
    beautiful — array.

But that's my problem, dear — not yours.
We digress.
Just let me give you a little advice — a few tips.
Single men don't drive station wagons, and children are the only people in today's world
who buy Aqua Velva — and they don't buy it for themselves.

Look at you —— you're young — so beautiful.
I'm not trying to meddle.
I can't and shouldn't arbitrate this part of your life.
It may seem old-fashioned of me — but please remember, dear —
that if your date isn't drinking because he's on some kind of medication ——
it's best to put "it" off for at least two weeks.

Believe me.
Mother knows best.

Ultimatum

Yes Arny, I know what it means.
Of course, I know what it means.
Oh, I'm sick of that, Arny.
I've had enough of it, Arny.
Do you hear?
I'm sick and tired of being treated like a moron, Arny.
You see, Arny — my brain functions.
It really does.
Inside this pretty little head of mine are five very active pounds
    of grey matter.
I have a B.A., Arny.
I went to university, Arny.
Do you remember that?
We met there.
I was an honours grad.
Remember?
Were you?
I know who wrote *The Republic*.
I know the difference between communism and socialism.
I know who Quisling was.
I know what DNA is, Arny.
And most of all?
I know that if you don't start giving my brain a little credit, Arny —
bad things are going to come your way, buster.
You see, I'm sick of being just a showcase.

I'm sick of being introduced to your friends as, "My little doll" or
    "My pretty little wife" —
and then having all your slimy business friends make their slimy
    little comments.
"Hey Arny, way to go."
"Hey Arny, what's she costing you?"
"Hey Arny, could I borrow her sometime?"
Like I'm a thing.
A pretty piece of fluff.
Well — I'm tired of being pretty for the boys, Arny.
I'm tired of being your idea of the perfect picture of femininity:
Beautiful with a closed mouth.
To be opened only when your little Hubert or Henry or
    Huckleberry —
or whatever you're calling it these days —
comes calling ——

And that's another thing.
Naming your weeny, Arny?
It's so juvenile.
So dumb.
It's so man-like.
What if women did it?

This is Larry —— *(Indicates right breast)*
Curly —— *(Indicates vagina)*
And Moe. *(Indicates left breast)*

Oh yeah?
Well, I *am* a pig.
A big fat pig.
In fact, to prove it to you and the rest of the world —
I'll tell you what I'm going to do.

The next time you give one of your tedious, please-give-me-a-
    promotion
cocktail parties, and let out one of your irritating "Isn't she
    wonderfuls?"
I'm going to turn to your boss, and fart.
It's going to knock the pictures off the neighbors' walls.
And then, Arny, I'm going to pick my nose, scratch my arm pits
    and burp.
And yes — they will call me a pig.
But at least I'll be something in their eyes other than your
    mannequin, Arny.
I'll have my own identity.
As a pig — but at least it will be mine.

Don't give me that shit, Arny.
I don't want to talk about it.

This One's Fur You

So there I was.
I reached out —— I felt it.
Oh, it was nice.
So soft — so very, very soft.
The woman beside me heard me whimper.
She smiled. She knew.
I took it off the rack.
I put it on.
I rubbed my cheek against it.
I started making little circles with my shoulders.
I made little moans like in foreplay.
"Oh, *mais oui.*"
Oh, I stroked it...
I ran my hands all over it.
Soon my shoulders were rolling and my hands were roving
　　all over the place.
Circular and angular — this way and that.
I was writhing and rocking — right there for everyone to see.
I didn't care.
I was free.
I was flying.
I was warm.
I was woman.
I was coming right there.
It was so good.
So real.

It was the decline and fall of everything moral.
All the pristine principles in my life were gone.
Everything naughty was made nice.
A cold wind blew inside me.
A sagebrush blew over my soul.
It was that good ——
And then I heard the first cry.
One tiny, pain-filled shrill.
Then another.
Then words — actual words.
"No — don't. I have children. They need me.
Think of my tiny little feet, and my little tail.
Think of my little nose as it catches scents in the air and darts
    all about.
So cute. I'm so cute. Please, please help me." ——
"Shut up."
I was at a crossroads.
My past was clashing with my present.
And I hate to clash —— you know that if you know me.
"Quiet," I said.
"Shut up. Don't give me this 60s crap. No more," I cried.
"No more of this flower-child, guilt-trip bullshit.
No more.
I won't listen."
I took a deep breath.
My shoulders started their circular motion again.
Soon my greedy, groping hands were all over it.
"Yes, yes, yes, yes..."
I'd faced it and won.
"Yeah, I'll take it — because I want it.
And the white fox as well.
Wrap them both.
I deserve it."

The Temptress

Oh no.
You can't love me.
No one can.
You're not good enough.
And you never will be.
However, I will also add, since I do feel quite sorry for you —
that another reason we can't pursue this sad little affair
is the fact that I am so very rotten.
It's true.
I am.
You just can't see it because you're so hopelessly enamored of me —
but I'm sure your friends have told you.

Take John, for example.
He wanted to live with me.
He begged me actually — on his knees.
Like a dog.
Grovelling.
Pleading.
Quite pathetic.
Swearing undying love.
He called me a goddess.
A work of art.
He read me Cohen.
Well I hate Cohen and just to shut him up I agreed to it on a
    trial weekend basis.

At 10 o'clock Saturday morning he fled from the house,
    left all his clothes
    and wasn't heard of again for two years —
    when he sent his mother a postcard
saying he had just moved in with his new lover — Jim —
and that he hated all women ——

And why?
Me.

So why don't you pack up your lovely intentions
and blind infatuation
and go bother someone else with them?
There are lots of women out there — not especially attractive
    or abundantly intelligent —
who would leap at the opportunity to have your charming
    schoolboy drool all over them.

Now, if you don't mind —
I have a lunch date to make this same speech to another sap.
Just like you.
Except this one likes Atwood.
How I hate Atwood.
The bitch.
God —— charm is a curse.

Uptown Girl

I find it very difficult to go back these days.

Yes, Tynam.
Yes.
Doubles.
Two.

I'll tell my boss I had double doubles and she'll warn me about
    too much caffeine.
I'm living in a different world than they are.
I am experiencing things that are simply not a part of their lives.
*(Sniffs and wipes nose with her fingers. This action used with
    discretion through piece.)*
I'm living the uptown way.
I'm 80s.
I'm today.
I'm early tomorrow for Chrissake.
And they couldn't be less impressed if they tried ——
Which I think they do.

I drop names left and right — all over the place.
"Pass the turkey — by the way, I met Al Waxman."
Yes, I did.
People, places, labels.
Like this: Alfred Sung.
Yes — now that's what I'm looking for.

That tiny intake of breath.
Just that thimble's worth.
Not a gasp — more a moan.
And that look on your face.
Appreciation of quality...envy.
That little longing to be just like me.
It's only natural —— I can handle it.
The bitchy modern woman — balls to her knees.
It's real.
I can touch it ——

But the folks back home...
Down to earth and then down just a little further.
I tell them where I've been ——
People I've rubbed shoulders with.
"Yes, that's right, I hang out at the same bar
      as the 20 Minute Workout gang.
You know: Muffy, Darla, Kiki, Lulu..."
What do I get?
Yawns, drifting attention, nail picking, crotch scratching.
They just don't know.
They think that working at Chateau is like working at K-Mart.
I'm just a check-out girl to them.
Oh, they're bitter, bitter people.
They're young — but they're trapped.
They're shackled to mortgages and kids.
The men are threatened by a woman who's making it in a world
that was supposed to belong to them.
And the women are jealous of the fact
that I can still give a man pleasure ——
Oh, I don't know...

Listen, I'm going to go powder my nose.
Care to join me?

ANDROGYNOUS

2

The Valedictorian

Good evening, ladies and gentlemen.

Yes, I'm getting ready ——
Get your tits off the ceiling.
I said my zits are peeling.
Everything grosses you out.

Ladies and gentlemen —
and those who wish their sexual ambiguities recognized ——
I celebrate your androgyny.
For all of us here tonight...our time has come.
I have been asked to speak tonight about our common bonds.
To touch your hearts.
To ennoble and edify you.
So that later as you writhe in the back seats of cars or in cheap
    motel rooms;
as you stoop over toilet bowls;
as you moon people down main street or pee on front lawns —
you will have something more to ponder than our treacle economy
and the hazards of unprotected fornication ——
In short, the black uncertainty that is the future.
That ominous place which only the aggregate of time can reveal.

I'll be two minutes —— so frig off.

What are the bonds?

What are those things that have made us one?
It was not this building.
It was not football, though we were football players —
    or debating, though we debated —
or the Theatre Club, though we were actors —
or the CB club, though we were ridden with acne
and somewhat strange to be with.
These were not the bonds, but the segregators.
What are they then? These bonds.
Masturbation — masturbation, I say, and bathroom going ——
The rest is man-made institution.
We came with it — we evacuate with it.
All else is social convention.

I'll be down in a second —— keep your thighs together.

I do not wish to be controversial.
I'm not sure I could.
Most of you who work here — except for you Mrs. Nickle
because you are 185 years old and were born a widow —
come from a generation that has robbed mine
of a fundamental right of all children:
to shock their elders.
You used foul language — deplored war — loved whales —
    cleaned up sex — drank like fish
and quite often — you abused drugs.
You have left us: teetotalism, vivisection, bigotry and virginity
as means of rebellion —— and it's just not worth it.
Conformity has become a beautiful thing.
We are a generation who ask only one thing:
Let us join your firm —— we want to buy things.

Two seconds — two bloody seconds.

But for the moment : the task at hand.
Tonight — the walls come tumbling down.
The world opens up.
Life the leveller — begins its work.
I descend this podium and at last I meet you.
Not as footballers, or debators, or thespians, or CBers ——
But as diddlers and shitters.
All in the same struggle — like we always were.
This is not the best age of man — but it is the best yet.
Peace to you all.

I — am —— coming.

Thank you.

The Existentialist

Ran over my own dog today.
Saw him ——
Could have stopped.
But why put off the inevitable?
I grabbed destiny by the wheel, and stepped on fate in the pedal
    — and said:
"No — this time I'm gonna get you. I'm one step ahead.
You sisters of fury three, weaving your threads —
I laugh at you. Ha.
Nay — I bark. Woof. No, bark I nay.
Ha.
You can't get me anymore. This guy's on to you."
When I got out of the car there was bird poop on the windshield.
I picked it up and put it on my shoulder — looking for pigeons
    to laugh at.
I couldn't find any — but I laughed all the same.
Ha.
I am the master now.

The sign says "Parking Any Time" ——
I slip a "No" in front of it.
In the dirt on my car, I write "Cops are Pigs".
I draw a big circle, and a smaller circle in it, and two smaller
    circles in it.
It's a pig as I see it and I love it.

Ha.
There's a lift in the crack of the sidewalk up ahead.
Nice try.
I see it. I choose it.
Smack ——
And it feels good.
My choice.
My decision.
No surprise.
No disappointment.
No anger ——
Just dirt all over my clothes and a smile on my puss.
Ha.

I went into work and I spit on my boss and I called her a bitch
and she fired me right on the spot.
Big deal.
I saw it coming — don't you see?
I make the decisions now.
Me.
When the baloney is green, I choose to eat it.
When the wine is red, I choose to spill it.
When the moment is all wrong — I choose it.
If I'm gutterbound —
If I'm sinking...down to the bottom —
then no one is going to take me there
but myself.
Get it?
Right on.
Right on.

A Hairowing Experience

It's always traumatic.
Of course, what isn't?
I avoid it as long as I can — but — I've got to have it done.
You want to live in civilization, you have to have your hair cut —
unless you want crowds of young men in studded leather
offering you drugs.
I don't ——
Most of the time I don't.
It's not the hair; I don't care about that.
It's where you have to go to get it done.
My ego can't take it.

The day I go to the hair stylist — I get up early — drink quite heavily
and leaf through *I'm O.K., You're O.K.* — feeling like hell.
I arrive — sweaty, very sweaty.
I give my name to an unimpressed receptionist.
"What would you like today?" ——
"I - I want my muffler changed. I want my hair cut —
and I want to get the hell out of here."
I'm told to take a seat.
I take a seat — lounge in some wicker — and sift through some
   old *GQs* —
which always make me wish I were dead.
I listen to the music and enjoy it — whether I like it or not.

And — I sit — and I wait — and I wait —
just long enough so that I know who's who in this world —
until, at last — the stylist bids me near.
I register how unimpressed he is —
but I realize that he does Carol Pope's hair
        and he's just doing me a favor.
I'm deeply honored.
Suddenly I'm having my hair washed by an unimpressed lackey
who I accept as a better person than me — and I deal with it.
I simply tell myself that I smell.

Then I suffer a great deal of embarrassment
        as I go from wash sink to cutting chair
with a towel wrapped around my head —
        looking like a damsel in distress
and wondering why when I describe myself I use feminine imagery.
I suffer a serious sexual identity crisis
as I try to explain what it is I want done to my head
to a person who probably suffers the same crisis all the time.
Moments later I realize that I have wasted my time and breath
as I watch myself in the mirror turn into The Thing from Planet V.

I also watch as my stylist's attention begins to wander
        to the window — the phone — the store.
I may be asked at some point what I do for a living —
but I know that the question is rhetorical because my answer
could never be as fascinating as — "Hairdresser".
At another point I'm told I have dandruff.
I watch The Thing from Planet V turn crimson.
Then I spot Carol Pope's autograph
and wish I were Carol Pope —— I really do.

I cry inside over the final result and agree with the stylist that
    he has done a wonderful job.
Then I cut off my left arm and leg — present them as payment
    — tip generously
and wish with all my heart and soul — that I were bald.

Somehow I'm just not very good at life.

A Canadian Blockbuster

Do I have it?
Do I have it?
Boy, do I have it.
It's current — it's topical — it's 80s — and best of all:
it reads, sounds and smells maple leaf.
This is Leonard Cohen singing "Ise the Bye" to Pierre Berton
      on Parliament Hill.
This is Anne Murray singing "Snow Bird" and eating back bacon
      on an Air Canada jet to Moose Jaw.
From now on we mount our shows — not the Canada Council.

OK. This is it.
It's 1930.
We pan to — keep ya hanging ——
To the prairies.
That's right.
Saskatchewan: flat — golden — golden with what?
Wheat.
Glorious Canadian wheat.
Then in the distance...but coming in closer — a barn.
A red barn.
A white farm house.
In the background music swells: Don Messer's Jubilee.
We only use Messer music.
We meet our central figure — a 16 year old — shuckin' corn or
      cuttin' wood.
One of those farm things.

The camera moves in and it stays there...for about 5 minutes.
It moves in on the sweat on his forehead — his arms — his legs.
Literally every part of his body.
Then — uh huh —
a train pulls up to a station — a prairie train station.
A well-dressed man steps off the train.
Louis James Skiffington LaFontaine.
The boy's uncle.
He has homes in Montreal and Toronto —— he's a business man.
You know the type.
He's come to convince the boy's father — his brother — to let
    him take the boy back east
and enrol him in Upper Canada College.

The kitchen —— the kitchen of the white farm house...
The boy comes in.
His father is sitting at the table.
The boy gives him a look —
a look that says, "I'm going to be better than you."

Like this.
Something like that.

The boy's mother is at the sink or stove.
We see her face. We move in on the wrinkles.
We need a face that tells stories — tired ——
We'll have to get a stage actress for that one.
She reaches up — to rub her breast — prescient — a little
    foreshadowing —
uh huh — that's right: breast cancer.
Not in a modern city with every facility imaginable...
No — this is circa depression prairies ——
Huh — is that not good.

The uncle arrives.
Everybody greets each other.
It's friendly...but not warm ——
There's something underneath.
Well the boy's father doesn't like his brother
and he doesn't want his son to go away.
He's an uneducated man — but no fool — uh huh.
He has soil savvy — which is our title, huh?
It's a pragmatism ——
A wisdom that can only come from toiling in good clean
    Canadian dirt.
The boy is anxious to leave, though.
He's impressed by the idea — and his uncle.

Before they leave — the boy, the uncle and the father go hunting
    in the bush.
Now there's probably not much hunting out there — but we'll
    film that in Ontario.
Anyway — the uncle takes all sorts of foolish risks with their lives
out there in the rugged Canadian Prairie Shield.
Finally he causes all three to break all six of their legs.
You with me?
OK. The Father makes them all splints and he builds a
    makeshift sled — huh?
It has now begun to snow.
If we can get a blizzard — better.
Now as they begin to trek back —
the uncle complains and indictates and wishes more than anything
that he was back in Toronto having lunch.

Suddenly — bears ——
Bears attack them.
They eat the food.

They eat the uncle.
They're not so bad.
To comfort the boy the father says the bears were only trying to
     protect and nourish their young.
The boy doesn't miss the parallel.
We don't miss the parallel.
Illiterates in Mozambique don't miss the parallel.
Images:
a father not wanting his son to leave —
a mother rubbing her breast —
and a father carrying his son the final 30 miles of their journey...

Denouement:
The boy learns respect and love for his father and his way of life.
He no longer yearns for the evil east.
He gains his soil savvy
and grows up to be the Premier of Saskatchewan.
But he never forgets that day.
I'm not sure if the mother should die...
I tell ya, kiddo ——
It's a winner.

The Actor

I was sitting alone.
Lonely.
Things had piled up.
Hadn't come together.
And then he came along.
The thing I needed the very least at that moment:
An actor.
I didn't want him to come, but he did.

Hey, you look down.
What's the matter?
Crash your Maserati into a tree?
Hey, did the — woman — give you a bad review?
Listen — she's done it to the best of us.
Done what?
It's too rude to say.
Hey, come on — her word isn't everything.
She's uptight.
Her last sexual experience was with a dinosaur.
Come on — the woman is a viper.
She'd give chicken bones to Lassie.

Would you please go away.
I don't think I'd like you even if I got to know you —
which is something I just don't want to do right now.

Work?
They talk about a theatrical slump, but it's been nonstop for this guy.
I just finished with a Wintario thing.
A one-man musical review of Hamlet.
I wrote it too.
Ya, I'm a writer.
But you could probably tell that.
I've got a writer's eye.

I kept telling him to go away but he wouldn't listen to me.
He didn't even notice me.
He didn't care.
The only thing he cared about was himself.
He never noticed anyone else.
If sheep could act, wolves would never go hungry
and you can quote me.

Hey — I've got an idea.
How about if I do some for ya?
Sure.
It'll make you feel better.
Got to be honest with ya.
They were mixed in Toronto, but they went crazy in Port Hope.
And they talk about Toronto sophisticates.

(Sings) To be or not to be
That is the big old question
Troubling me

Oh — hey.
Guess I could come up with a better one than that.
I've got it.

The end of the first-act grand finale.
I usually have a tambourine.

Get thee to a nunnery.
Get thee to a nunnery.
Please get out of here.
We don't want ya here.
Your hair is messy,
Your clothes are funny,
And your breath smells
Like you just ate
A big bag of fertilizer.
And you've got
No sense of humor.
You're such a downer.
Get thee to a nunnery.
I don't know what
They'll do to you there,
But maybe Ophelia. (oh-feel-ya)
But baby you're so
Very svelte. Don't forget
Your chastity belt.
And take an extra key
In case you lose one
And go crazy out of your mind
Trying to find it.
Get thee to a nunnery.
Ya!

He was gone and I was glad.

Overdue

I checked under my arms to confirm what I already knew.
Two dark patches forming at the top of my sleeves.
I put my nose to my shoulder, pretending to scratch —
    actually trying to smell.
I saw a lady look at me and give me a little benign smirk.
She had two dark patches too.
Commiseration, I thought, is one of life's greatest comforts.

I was about fifth in line at the counter.
Everyone in front of me seemed to have about fifteen books each.
"Unemployed," I thought.
I guess my face must have read a benign little smirk too —
here was more comfort.
Their pits were dry though ——
You can't have everything.
With that many people and those many books it took a while.
The elderly lady behind the counter was doing her best —
though you could see she couldn't wait for the economy to pick up.

With all this time, my mind had a chance to further flagellate itself ——
My library daymare started again.
I'd reach the front of the line — an ancient hand would reach out
and take my card, checking my name and my face.
One of her pencilled-in eyebrows would rise ——

Her withered lips would slam together ——
And everyone else at the counter would hear a malignant "Hmmm!"
"Uh — Uh — what's wrong, Miss?"
"Perhaps you can tell me?"
"Ah — I don't know."
"I think you do. Aren't you the same man who took out *1984*
     over two months ago —
the same man who received countless letters from us requesting
     one thing:
the return of our book.
How can you be so selfish?"
"I - I - I'm sor——"
"I bet you are. Guard! We have been watching you ——
And we have been waiting."

The guard —— he drags me to the basement.
Oh, it's awful.
A horrible place.
Damp and dirty and smelly.
Remnants of human beings crawl around dragging balls and
     chains behind them.
One of them shuffles over to me and says:
"I'm doing two months for *The Great Code*; I left it at the beach."
Another human leftover yells out, "*The National Dream* — eight
     weeks."
And then the door swings open, and a deep voice says, "Rations,"
and throws them into the pit.
All the human crumbs run to it —
tearing, ripping, kicking and biting each other.
The man in for *The Great Code* comes over to me — blood all
     over his teeth and feet — and he says:
"I got pages 120-156 of *Surfacing*. You better get over there fast.
     There might be some prelims left —— Hurry!"

It's mayhem.
People literally gorging themselves.
A *Readers Digest* whizzes past.
"Care for an hors-d'oeuvre?" someone shouts.
No.
It's horrible.

I tried to get away.
I turned — I turned again.
I turned here — I turned there —
I just ran ——
And suddenly there were little books at my feet ——
Yes, it's true.
Their covers were opening and they were screaming:
"Read me, read me, read me or we'll be sent to the stacks...
Fish tales and cooking books — no — no.
We'll be remaindered."
"Remainder," someone cries out —— damned near killed her.
"No," I cry, "no" ——
And I fall to the floor — the little pages flapping all around me ——
"Read me, read me!"

Suddenly, though, I hear an old woman's voice saying,
"Thank you sir, have a nice day."
She's handing me my books ——
Checked out.
I'm free to leave.
I've bucked the system — again.
Life is full of triumphs.

To The Avid Theatregoer

The avid theatregoer is a member
of that ever burgeoning facet of our society
which regularly attends a theatrical event.
In the outer reaches of our province he is a ticket holder to one
      of our many and increasingly important regional theatres.
And in the metropolitan areas of our nation
he is a viewer perhaps of a touring Broadway production
or one of those experimental things.

The avid theatregoer almost always begins his evening dining out...
Tonight he is on his way to a charming little French restaurant
He heard about from a friend.

They arrive — greet the maitre d' — peruse the surroundings ——
Yes, this will do.
This will do just fine.
Dinner: French onion soup, a cheese crêpe of some sort,
for dessert something sinfully caloric
and — of course — almond blackberry tea.
All downed with a little white wine, a domestic thing — and a
      lime perrier chaser.
Just enough to make them both a little silly.
With dinner done — tummies filled, palates satisfied — they're off —
with just a hint of schoolgirl anticipation
to — yes —— the theatre.

After a somewhat intensive search they find a parking spot and
    begin their hike
to — yes —— the theatre.
They arrive — check their coats — take their seats...
While they wait his date reminds him just once more that
    she had drinks one time with three of the cast members.
Oh really, he rejoins ——
Then suddenly — the theatre doors close.
The house lights lower...
They lean forward in their seats
as the curtain rises on the proscenium of the stage
and the play begins to unfold before the audience.

Three tedious hours later our theatregoer is still there.
Crammed into those ridiculously small seats —
    his little bottom all sweaty.
Hoping beyond hope
that this completely incomprehensible piece of trash
will end and end now.
Finally.
At last.
The curtain falls.

Soon they're shuffling their way up the aisle
with a gnawing, pecking feeling at the back of their necks.
The one you get when you know you've wasted your time and
    money.
At last — finally — they reach the coat check
Where they wait for twenty minutes
while a somewhat overweight, acne-ridden, pregnant young lady
    says to them:
"Listen pal, you think you got problems."

At last they receive their coats, and as they turn,
        who but who do they meet
but that stupid idiot from their night course at the university.
The single most opinionated person ever created.
He offers up all his unwanted opinions
about every aspect of this evening's performance ——

"Oh, it was marvelous — it was wonderful — it was real —
it was multi-leveled — it was Ibsenesque ——"
It was crap.
And our theatregoer is perfectly aware of it.
After twenty minutes — and only to catch his breath —
this idiot turns to our theatregoer and says ——
"So what did you think of it?"
Well, what is he to do?
If he says he didn't like it he'll have to defend his opinion —
which of course he can't do ——
Because he didn't understand a damn thing after the curtain went up.
He'll have to lie — fabricate — bullshit his way out of this one.
Like he's never done before.
If you didn't understand it — just say you loved it.
Which is exactly what he does.
He looks this man straight in the eyes and says ——
"I thought it was the single most important theatrical event
to hit this town in five years.
I'm seeing it again."

And he does.
God bless him.
And Toto too.

It's My Funeral And I'll Plan It If I Want To

You're not watching your game.
Look what you're about to do.
OK — go ahead. Pardon me.
Check.
I tried.

You know, I heard three people say that he looked asleep —
and not cynically ——
I didn't know people still said that.
I didn't know people in the 80s could be that maudlin.
I would hate it ——

(Referring to the game) Don't do that.

I look like hell when I'm asleep.
I don't want them to say I look asleep.
I want them to say:
"He looks like he's sailing on a warm August night."
I want to be a corpse of whom it can be said, "It was sexy." ——

Don't do that.

After all, the body is the temple of the Lord.
And mine's the Acropolis ——

Don't do that.

Don't do that —— you're doing it.
Check.

If you want to go out with the garbage — fine.
The Man from Glad as your funeral director ——
It's OK with me.
It's money in the bank.
I'm going in a big way.

A church service? I'll need it.
Church meaning cathedral — with a priest — meaning bishop.
Preferably Rome's ——

Don't do that.

Dress code? Formal and black.
Black — black — black —— short of shoe polishing your faces
and hiring the Globetrotters as pallbearers.

Do you want some more cookies? Tea? Anything? ——

Don't do that.

The eulogy. Well, the Queen. Who else?
The head of state — our tear-filled Queen
spouting nothing but lies.
And an attitude should be adopted.
An air of mass hysteria — mixed with deep depression.
Gigglers should be shot, dry eyes soaped.
And — afterwards — a gathering ——

Check.

Something somber. No alcohol — no party.
All in whispers.
As activities...maybe slide shows with a narration of my life.
Pool, blackjack, casino wheels, white elephant tables?

No.
No way.

Insouciant guitar accompanied renditions
of "Kum-Ba-Ya" and "Blowing in In the Wind" —
    in three-part harmony.

Sure — yes, of course.
Slamdancing, nosers, group massages, videos, tupperwear
and Shakely vitamin selling?
Tacky.
Really tacky.
Fainting, wailing, human sacrifices?
Of course.
And then maybe each year on the day of my demise —
till — oh, the end of time —
a small candlelight vigil on Parliament Hill.
For the grieving throngs to remember and weep.

Checkmate.

Cookie? ——

Opal

Oh, I don't know, Cin.
I look around and I see that whole wicker, hanging plants thing.
That whole 70s craze:
Blondie, punk parties — that whole New Wave thing —
and I think, "It's yesterday —— it was nice but it's over."
I just don't know what to say.
I'd hate to be arbitrary and say peach and black, but at this point ——

Good morning. Le Bon Homme.
May I help you?
Yes.
Well, I'm sorry, we have nothing until two. Yes, OK...
No, I'm sorry — nothing till two.
Do you want me to put you down for then?
Sure — of course, alright. That's fine.
No, I don't need it — that's two o'clock today. See you then ——
No, I'm sorry. Sale prices till Wednesday only —— thank you — bye.

Larry, aging butch number for two.

(Sings) Gonna wash that gray right out of his hair.
Oh get over it.
You're soaking in it.
But Madge — I thought Palmolive was green.

Oh my goodness.
Who is that.

Robert, is that your 11:30?

Not anymore.
Take a break, honey.
Do something useful.

Well, hello.
My name is Opal.
I'm your stylist for today.
Please walk this way.
This is Cinnamon.
He's sometimes our wash girl.
Oh get over it, girl.
Sorry — we're just a little crazy around here.

Can we talk.
How about that Joan?
What a bitch, eh?
What you're wearing today is a very unique combination.
Don't get me wrong, I like it ——
It's sort of a Le Chateau Lumberjack.

Now let's just feel this, see what we're dealing with.
Holy Mother Marilyn.
This hair is dead.
D.E.D. dead.
Straw.
Horse food, honey.
Don't tell me —— I know your type.
The only cream rinse you use is water
and a split end is what you sit on.
Right?

Girls, girls — Larry, Robert, come here —
Ensemble, ensemble.
Feel this. Oh oh, it's hair tragedy. Look — girls, girls ——
Quiet.
I am an artist, and hair is the canvas that I paint on ——
And I can't deal with this.

Well — just because I cut hair doesn't mean ——
Well you just take your lovely little hind end out of my shop.
Get out.

Oh Cin, did you hear him.
Oh, I'm so flustered.
I need a tea.
I need a peppermint tea and I need it now.
Get me my amyl.

Oh, I don't know, Cin — what do you think of mauve?

Party

I'll never do it again.
It was awful.
Just dreadful.
An unmitigated social disaster.
Everyone wanted out.
I wanted out.
Never mind not getting off the ground ——
This baby dug a hole — a trough — a ditch —
a canal of Welland proportions.
A giant festive egg was laid here tonight and I was the conduit.
It was the party from hell —— and I hosted.
I'll never be forgiven.
I don't want to be.
I don't deserve it.
In a more sophisticated world, what I gave tonight would be a
    capital offense.
I'll be a pariah for years.
Yes, it's that serious.
I raped 63 people of their Saturday night.
I killed it.
It was merciless.
We're talking charades by 8:30.
Trivial Pursuit at 9:00.
By 9:30, people were ripping down all my "No Dinking In Here" signs
and humping anything that moved — their worst enemy —
Just to have something to do.

It was a massive orgy of contempt.
A giant oinkarama of hate.
I bet the sex was great ——

Conversation died tonight.
And we buried it.
And not decently.
Nothing clicked.
It didn't even ick.
The theme thing was a bust. It always is.
The beach, the 50s, the 60s, the 70s; it doesn't matter what.
It could be your favorite food group.
The gays came in dresses — the hets in bathing suits.
Doug, the sex beast, wore a Speedo and a tank top —
throwing one third of the guests into expectorant hypertension
following the Great Dangler wherever it went.
At one point, we had 24 people in the bathroom, knee-deep in drool.
Thankfully, all he'd done was drink all day.
I couldn't wait to get out of there.

Four art students held the great debate in the living room
over something I bought at Woolco ——
A barf-wrenching display that forced huge numbers of guests
    into the kitchen
where a disproportionate number of people
started eating disproportionate amounts of food —
so that by 8:45 there was a minor scuffle over some cheesy crumbs.
Somewhere in there a certain fashion designer I know
spilled an entire bottle of amyl nitrate on the floor —
sending the guests dancing in that room into a frenetic fit
that I thought would bring the house down.

One ordinarily demure young thing (so I'm told) began shouting ——
"Yes baby — oh baby, do it."
She has since called to apologize and ask if I know where to
     get the stuff.
"Sure baby, headshops and gay bars ——
Maybe you need some condoms, a little hooch maybe?"
What is this? ——
Cindy's Sex Aids?
Oh yeah, then the same fashion designer was at the center of a
     short scratch fight
after he likened lovemaking to one of the guests
as "pumping the pudding."
He's off my party lists.

Actually, that's a kindness ——
I'll keep him on.

By this time it's all of 10:30 and Bread's *Greatest Hits* is
     already on the turntable.
Tapestry is out of its jacket, set to go next.
I can still hear one certain fashion designer howling,
"You make me feel like a natural woman."
The pooning has abated.
The jam session on the front porch is over ——
No more American Pie.
The back porch cry-and-counselling area for fights
between this bitch and that prick with best friend referees
     has cleared.
Three-quarters of the guests are gone by 11:00 ——
All of them the interesting ones.
Those remaining I don't know and are legally brain dead
or marvelling at their hands or the lamps or the color green —
laughing intermittently and asking, "Has Jim gone?" ——

Jim is that enigmatic figure who deals in drugs —
walking neighborhood streets, listening for loud music —
    looking for cramped driveways —
finally sticking his head in the front door
and naively asking any one of the 42 people in the foyer:
"Is there a party, man?" ——
He's sort of an updated mask of death.

By 12:00, the local bars are knowing unusually good business ——
And the party's over.
It's just me and my tears, scraping wax off the coffee table —
a man in a pantsuit screeching, "It's too late baby" —
and Jim on my bed in a coma.

Never ——
Never ever again.
Uh uh.
No way.
The end.

Male

3

Funny Goy

When I was a kid, I wanted to be a comic when I grew up.
But I got off to a bad start.
Not black, not Jewish.
What chance did I have?
See, people in those groups have got it made.
Oppression.
You want to be funny — you've got to have it.
It produces either terrorism or standup comedy.
I wonder if you can be both.
A funny terrorist, hmmm.
"Don't anybody move or I'll blow your fucking heads off."
Just kidding. *(Imitates machine gun fire)*
Don't ever trust anyone with a machine gun."
See, everything about minority groups is a seed for humor:
their family relationships, the struggle to be accepted but to
    retain tradition ——
Now that is very funny stuff.
Even their food:
Gefilte fish —— that is a very funny food.
When was the last time you heard a gut splitter about Yorkshire
    pudding? ——
And you never will.

My family: not a very amusing institution.
Well, we have one mildly funny event every year.

My grandmother —— she's old and you know form follows function
so every Christmas there's a fight over who has to sit beside her.
I don't know — the food, the excitement ——
Everyone's talking down the table ——
"How are you?" "What's new?" "Funny joke — haha —"
and then — at Granny's end — the conversation starts to die
and the silence works its way down the table...
Uh, uh, ooh.
In the fish tank, they're diving for the bottom.
The corners of the wall paper are curling and the centre piece is
        wilting
and you know that if you're going to survive
you have exactly three seconds to get-the-fuck out of there ——
My family.
Nice, pleasant — but boring.
Muzak incarnate.
And me — I was such a normal kid it was pathetic.
A confirmed heterosexual by 3.
A member of the Young Conservatives by 8 ——
Damned normality.

There was a guy, though, who lived on our street.
Now there was a funny guy.
Horrible family.
Low grade.
His parents — little education, poor hygiene.
As a baby, he caught hoof-and-mouth disease from breast feeding.
But he was funny ——
Or maybe lucky.
See, very early on he discovered that the only thing it takes
to make a 10-year-old convulse with laughter
is the word "boner."

And in our neighborhood, it was his word.
No one else touched it.
It was his in for every pre-pubescent social function on the block.
But then in grade 8 — life turned on him.
It was a May day.
May 10th, 1971.
I don't know why I remember, but I do.
It was the day of his Waterloo.
It was his Gettysburg.
It was his Winnipeg Convention.
It was a health class.
Not mental health — not for him, not for any of us...

The teacher turns the lights out and the projector on.
Multi-colored cartoon sperm and ovaries dance across the
      screen.
"The Blue Danube" in the background.
(Whistles this and imitates the sperm with his index finger)
The sperm assemble — little rocket jets strapped to their backs.
It's seconds before launch.
The countdown begins.
10 — 9 — 8 ——
Then a big booming deep voice comes on: "This is an erection."
And he explains it.
Everyone looks at Mike — that was his name.
The word boner was dead.
They'd made it clean.
It wasn't funny anymore.
Poor guy.

My family moved — but years later I heard Mike had a nervous
    breakdown in grade 10.
Latin again —— goddang Latin.
Fellatio, fornication...
What disgusting words.
They got him again.
Sad story.

They'll get ya coming.
They'll get ya going.

The One And Only

I think there's only one perfect match for each of us ——
Our soul mate.
One special person with our name written all over them.
That's it.
The sad part is that most of us never meet her.
She's out there but you never know where.
I'd been married for four years and I still didn't know where mine was.
Eventually you have to settle for second best.
A reasonable facsimile is what 90% of mankind sleeps next to.
It's not such a terrible thing.
Imagine the meaningless futility of life
if you didn't have anybody to watch TV with.
Somebody to yell at.
Somebody you don't have to be interesting with.
You spend your time with the best you can find — at the
    moment ——
Which is where we all live.
So her image isn't occupying every cell in your brain;
so she's not constantly coming up with insights that you thought
    only you ever thought of;
so she doesn't fart publicly and your parents love her.
It's give and take.
Magic's for the movies.
I know.
'Cause I met my one and only.
She just walked into my life.

It was incredible.

God existed —— and He was good.

My soul mate and I were the same species and the opposite sex ——

Which is, of course, not always the case.

She was exquisite.

Ugly as sin : the woman could make barf throw up.

But I saw her in different way.

I didn't see her as fat —— she was full.

In fact she was spilling all over the place.

But who cared.

She was beautiful.

She spoke to me.

You know what I mean?

Everything she did or said talked to me.

"Yes, yes," I always wanted to say to her, "that's the way I think ——

That's the way I see things too."

The way she looked at people and art and food and nefariously
     immoral sex acts ——

God love her.

We just became the best of friends: two young teenaged girls.

I'd tell her what I was going to wear. We'd giggle.

And we'd talk in baby garble.

We threw out consonants. We sounded like smurfs:

I wuv you —— I wuv you too.

I wuv you this much ——

I wuv you even more.

And then one day ——

One day...

We were going to go on a romantic winter walk.

I told my wife I was going to the driving range.

There was three feet of snow. I don't even golf! ——

My wife is so dumb.

I went to the place where we were supposed to meet —

and I waited and waited.
The things that went through my mind in an hour — waiting,
    waiting ——
And finally I saw her.
I got all excited.
I was like a puppy dog.
My tail was wagging and I had this huge grin on my face.
I started to yell —— I called her name:
"Bertha, Bertha I wuv you, I wuv you."
She started across the street and she didn't see it coming ——
A Honda Civic.
Such a small car. Such a big woman.
She flew.
She did 60 easily —— just off into the distance.
"I wuv you ——
I weally, weally do."

The Goof

Just wait — before you tell me.
I want you to know — that whatever —— I've given this a lot of thought.
I mean — I've gone over it a thousand times.
I've racked and banged my brains.
I've really abused my mind over this one.
And I want to tell you — before you tell me —
so that later if the answer is "No"
then you'll know I'm not just making cheap promises like I might
    have done.
Because that's always the easy thing to do.

Got it? —— good.

I want you to know — that I'll be beside you.
I'll — I'll stand by your side.
I know it sounds like an old song — but I'll do it.
I mean — I would rather not have to. I'd rather the answer was "No."
A beautiful bouncing baby "no" ——
'Cause I have plans...
And nowhere in my great scheme of things is the word "Pampers."
No — you just don't know how many times I've seen young guys
    with party-girl wives ——
A stroller in one and a JVC in the other.
I think: "There, but by the grace of withdrawal, go I."

It scares me.
It's a very messy thought, if you know what I mean.
It's a dark day for the Fruit of the Loom ——
I want you to know that.

I'm young.
I'm way too young ——
despite what the birth certificate says —
I'm still a baby.
And babies should not beget babies.
My mother did — and look at the result.
It's a job for adults — and if I stay on the course I'm on now
I'm not going to be one until I'm well over 50.
Which is probably pretty common.
Just confirming that I am Joe Ordinary.
A common everyday guy ——
God — our kids will be ugly.
But I want you to know —— I want to comfort you.
I want to help —— I'll get a job.
I'll quit school and I'll get a job.
Oh God, I hate to work —— a few weeks in the summer — if I
    really have to.
But I've got no skills.
I can't do anything.
The only thing I do well is nothing.
You don't know how many times I've prayed that this is a glitch.
Since the faucet stopped leaking —
since the sparrows didn't come home to Capistrano ——
I've been on my knees — forty times a day — begging the
    maker of the universe
that on that stupid night I had a sperm count of 6.
Six tailless, toothless, tadpoles with no sense of direction —

and no desire to be anything more than they already were.
But I'll do it.
I'll do the honorable thing.
I'd rather be a sleaze bag.
A creep and a prick ——
But I won't.
You've got my word.
My feeble little word.
That's all I'm going to say.
It's your turn.

I can't.
I can't listen.
I don't want to know ——
Who am I kidding?
So I'm a sleaze bag.
I can live with that.
Look, on the one hand — let's say my left —
I'm faced with being the biggest prick of the century.
And on the other hand — the right hand —
I see smelly diapers and a job at GM.
And I gotta tell ya —— I'm going for the left.
And now I'm going for the door.
I may be a prick — but I'm a single prick.

Later.

Malcolm

His story wasn't about regained sight or healed limbs.
About people pulling through or bad ones becoming nice ones.
His always seemed hopeless.
Malcolm was small.
His body was.
His apartment was.
His job was.
His conversation was.
Everything about him seemed underdeveloped.
Malnourished.
Lacking something.
Those who knew him called him a wimp.
They were right.
It's not that he was effeminate.
Even faggots used to call Malcolm a wimp.
'Cause he was.
Then he went to the dentist.
He was sure to do that every six months.
He was afraid of tooth decay.
Really afraid.
He picked up a magazine.
And read it.
Hunters World.
And he bought his own.
He read it.
From cover to cover.

Story after story about men and guns.
And the animals they kill with their guns.
In the great outdoors.
Man, the elements, nature's wild children and ammo.
Raw conflict.
Them or you.
Survival of the fittest.
It made Malcolm hard.
He never got hard.
Who'd fuck him if he did?
He bought more magazines.
Books.
Then he bought a gun.
A license.
He bought new boots.
New hunting wear.
A tent.
Every piece of gear he might ever need, Malcolm bought.
He bought the best.
He looked the part.
He liked what he saw and he felt good.
Something new for Malcolm.
He packed the car and headed north.
Where the animals live.
He drove fast.
He drove sometimes past the speed limit.
He never did that before.
Malcolm was changing.

He reaches the north and he unpacks his sack.
He locks the car and heads into the woods.
He walks and walks.

It's hot.
Sweat pours down his face.
He never sweats.
Mosquitoes circle him but don't bother him — or with him.
For hours he hikes.
Never stopping.
Filled with the forest.
Then, at last, the sun begins its sluggish summer set.
Malcolm makes his camp.
Sets up his tent.
Builds his fire.
Cooks his meal.
Underneath the sky.
The sounds of day turn into the sounds of night.
A haunting chorus rises around him. To him it's the most
    beautiful tune ever played.
He is truly alone.
Lesser men would be frightened.
Not Malcolm.
He dreams no dreams that night.
He spent the day — dreaming.
When morning comes he's ready.
A hunter ready to hunt.
He knows the signs to look for.
The broken branches.
The chewed leaves.
The pooh.
And soon he's on to something.
The Minotaur in his maze.
The day takes him miles and miles into the woods.
It brings him closer and closer to his chase.
Each step takes him closer to something great.
He can feel it.

Taste it.
And then it's there.
A deer.
A young deer.
He sees the animal and the animal sees him back.
It seems tired.
Resigned.
It doesn't move.
You see — it knows.
It knows why Malcolm has come.
Malcolm raises his gun.
He cocks it.
His mind is filled.
Millions of synopses charged.
In it he sees a deer.
A killer, with fangs, with poison.
Tearing flesh.
Cruel and calculating
No.
No pity.
Deserving to die.
And then there is the deer that stands before him.
He points his gun.
He waits.
Shoot.
Wait.
Shoot.
Wait.
Shoot damn it —— shoot!
He shoots.
He yells.
He screams.
Go.

Run.
Run, you fucker, run.
And somewhere above the trees
the bullet tilts back to the earth — and falls.
A harmless empty shell.
Malcolm smiles.
Not a polite smile.
Not an ingratiating smile.
Not a required smile.
Back to his car.
Back to the city.
Different though.
Very different.

And back here, doctor — to finish.
I won't be back again.
I've outgrown you.
You will be happy to know that I no longer need you.
50 minutes, doctor.

All done.

Bible Minute Bob

Hello boys and girls.
I'm Bible Minute Bob and it's time for another Bible Minute.

Last week we left off with our home question:
"What happens to little boys and girls who ask questions like:
"If there were dinosaurs, why doesn't the Bible mention them?"
Well, little Davey Gardner of Kenora, Ontario knows.
He writes: "Why, they go to hell — where the intense heat
    causes their skin to burn
and singe in terrible, wretched pain for all eternity."
Very good, little Davey Gardner of Kenora, Ontario.
This week our Bible Minute T-Shirt goes out to you.

Now, last week we learned that God —
after many failed attempts at creating companionship with:
Homo Pithicus —— too ugly;
Homo Erectus —— too stupid;
and the Neanderthal —— too testy —
had settled on Homo Sapiens.
You and me.
And the first two editions were called Adam and Eve.
Well, this week we learn that Adam and Eve lived in a place
called the Garden of Eden.
Here they were allowed to romp about without cares and without
    clothes.

That's right, boys and girls, they were naked and they didn't have
    to work.
Some people, called theologians, call this Paradise.
Others have a different name for a forest
where people romp about in perpetual unemployment ——
They call it Newfoundland.

Till next week, boys and girls — our home question is:
"What happens to little boys and girls who grow up to like little
    boys and girls?"
I'm Bible Minute Bob ——
God bless.

Reconciliation

I don't do it that way.
I don't like the one on one method.
It's too difficult.
I go to group confession.
The church offers it once a year for people like me.
It's a mass.
A priest reads a list of general sins
and you mentally check off which ones you're guilty of —
and you feel bad about them.
It's still difficult, though.
The church is more lax now, but if this were 20 years ago...
During the last year I've probably chalked up the penance equivalent
of 14 million Hail Marys.
Which breaks down to: 5 or 6 for every drunk, 1 or 2 for swearing,
20 or 30 for saying bad things about my mother,
and about 150 per sexual act.
Three hundred if you shared the experience ——
And this year people were very generous.

I arrive at church one very sweaty, nervous, depraved creature.
The first thing I notice is the incense ——
It smells so nice but it makes you feel just awful.
I cautiously approach the holy water font — slowly, tenuously
    dipping my fingers,
threads of Dracula spinning in my mind ——

It's cold.
Father, Son and the Holy Spirit — amen ——
Thank you.
Then into the church.
Packed.
There are lots of me.
I take the only seat I can find.
I'm the youngest in our pew — by 92 years.
As I sit down they all look at me: sagging cheeks, dangling
    chins, pursed lips ——
A sinner has arrived and they know it.
Then the priest comes out and the litany of sins begins.
Drinking is not a sin — lest it be in excess.
What other kind of drinking is there?
And on and on he goes — sin after sin ——
And it's me.
It's all me.
This man's been living in my pants.
Finally the end of the list.
The climax:
Sex.
My face turns a very tell-tale beet red.
I turn to my left ——
Four pairs of cataracts pointed right at me.
Jealous?
And all around the hallowed floors are littered
with Catholic on Catholic — writhing in guilt.
People on the edge of pews.
Tears pouring down their faces.
But then — at last:
The priest.
This venerable representative
of the 2000-year-old uninterrupted apostolic succession

established by the Son of God himself — sorry but I am a
    Catholic after all —
raises his hands and says: "You are forgiven."
It's OK.
Ah, shit — do you feel good.
And you know that your soul is clean and pressed and ready to go.
Go and have one very large, very well-deserved drink
or two or three or four...

I wouldn't be anything but a Catholic.

Caught In The Act

I wondered how long it would take you, but I never imagined
    you'd be this quick ——
You're good, Mary.
I guess I didn't know how good.
You're absolutely right, of course.
I didn't go bowling tonight.
No, no — I didn't.
As a matter of fact I've never been bowling, Mary.
I wouldn't know a 10 pin from a 5 pin if they rolled over my face.
I think bowling is ludicrous.
I don't have the belly for it.
I've got all my hair.
I'm not built for it, Mary ——
No, no — let me explain; you deserve the truth.
The trophies I get each year I buy myself.
I try to be modest.
I try to figure out what would be an accurate reflection of my
    bowling ability —
which is strictly unrealized potential.
That's why they keep getting bigger.
I figure I'd just keep getting better.
I'd get some technique — I'd work in my shoes —
and I'd learn to spit — spit like a bowler should.
On anything, on anyone — for the game.
And so of course you realize —— let me finish —
that the bowling banquets were all a lie too.

I was going to start pushing it this year by introducing the
    Bowling Retreat Weekend.
Just some quiet time — you know Mary — for me and my ball
to be together — alone — in the mountains.
One on one, in a way that I'd really rather not discuss.

You should also know, Mary, that I didn't actually go to McGill.
I know someone who did and I stole his jacket.
He was my size and that's what our friendship was based on.
I really only went to George Brown, "the City College."
I was going to be a cake decorator ——
That's when I changed my name.
Mom and Dad were Nazis, Mary. I'm not really Irish.
It was shortly after that that I started to do the drag shows.
Where am I when I'm supposed to be bowling, Mary? ——
I'm in a downtown bar mouthing the words to "The Way We Were"
in a full-length Christian Dior.
I do Tina, Donna, Bette and Barb.
I do them all —— and I'm good.

You see, growing up as a young woman in Paraguay I discovered
    that my true self
was actually a man — you can understand that — and so I took
    the steps
to actualize who I really was — to validate myself as a person.
But years of feminine engendering stuck with me.
It needed an outlet — and the stage was there.
Of course, it wasn't till many years later that I met Peter
and discovered that although once a woman, then a man — I
    was now gay.
Peter and I are still together ——

We keep a small apartment and we plan to adopt children.
We're very happy together.

Now, I could stay here and tell you more —
about the drugs and prison and the whole thing —
but Peter and I are going shopping —
I need some nylons ——
And later on we're going dancing.

I'm sorry I'm late, Mary.
What can I say?

Summer Blahs

Perhaps there's something wrong in not wanting to have the
    complexion
of a Tibetan sheepherder by the time I'm 40? ——
I don't think so.
Unlike the rest of this nation,
simply because the calendar tells me it's summer,
I see no need to strip naked, go outdoors and go quite literally
    out of my mind for 4 months.
I'm quite, quite happy indoors, thank you.
Where, by the way, human beings belong.
I see no grave mental disorder in not wanting to grease my
body like a rear axle and go to a beach
with a higher bacteria count than a pair of trucker's underwear
to catch a Frisbee with my big toe.
Under all the definitions I have of what constitutes a good time,
the word "Frisbee" never appears.
Not even once.
Grease — alright, a few times — but that's not the point.
I have more important things to do.

Call me a tight ass.
I'll only take it as a compliment.
Look — maybe if I had a body that could elicit comments like:
"Wow, what a tan!" or "Hey, nice pecs!" instead of, "I see your
    stomach and breasts have gone south for the summer,"
or, "Hey pal, better get some Noxema on that."

So just stop making me feel guilty because I'm not having the
    time of my life —
and I suppose that's the crux...
I resent the fact that simply because it's too hot for a jacket I'm
    expected to have a good time.
I can barely stand having a good time when it's spontaneous ——
It's unbearable when it's forced on me.

Summer — for me — is like one giant perpetual baby's birthday
    party.
The baby doesn't know what's going on.
It doesn't know how to "party."
In fact, it's having a lousy time.
It wants to be in its crib sucking on its feet.
It doesn't want to be propped up in a high chair, wearing a
    ridiculous hat
and having 10 drunk adults who'd rather be somewhere else
sing a lousy round of "Happy Birthday" —
and then force fed lousy cake and ginger ale.
No adult would stand for it.
You see, if only this poor little exploited piece of humanity
had a voice, it would say ——
"Mom, Dad, Grandma — piss off. All of you just go home.
Go make love. Go read a book. But leave me alone.
All I want to do is stay in my crib
and suck on my feet and pooh in my pants."
In the summer — I'm the same way:
I want to stay in my crib and suck on my feet.

You go to the beach.

Lunch With Jean-Jacques

Jean-Jacques and I met as teenage boys
while attending the same exclusive private school in Canada.
None of the royal family ever went there.
It was that exclusive.
Jean, by the by, was French.
He was from France.
As are millions of other people.
We had been such good friends.
We contrasted each other perfectly.
I was slight and pleasant looking.
He was rugged and handsome.
I was intelligent and witty.
He was more intelligent and more witty.
I was well liked.
He was worshipped.
I was well-endowed.
He would make tracks in the sand like a Massey Ferguson plough.
Our friendship flourished.
By this time, I hadn't seen him for a number of years.
He'd gone back to Paris after school.
I had heard, through the vin de grape, that he had recently fallen
    on hard times —
and I was anxious to see for myself.
I caught a Concord in New York.
I'm forever catching something in New York.
Nice place to visit — but don't touch.

Anyway — the flight was a delight.
And, if I may — so was the syntax of that last sentence.
I sat beside a charming nuclear physicist from Denver
who couldn't pronounce his R's or his T's, Q's, E's, A's, L's
his Z's, M's, N's, O's, D's and sometimes Y.
It was at times difficult to understand what he was saying.
It must cause him a lot of hardship —
but of course I pretended not to notice ——
I've dealt with the handicapped.
Recently, I've learned that the Chinese word for Peking
sounds remarkably like the word Denver.
Perhaps — who knows?
Anyway, I arrived safely in Paris — my beautiful Ville d'illumine.
Going to Paris is for me a social orgasm.
After a lovely but exhausting evening at my hotel — what a fine
    young staff they have —
I was up at ten the next morning,
very anxious about my lunch date with Jean-Jacques that day at two.
I had planned for weeks what I would wear and wasted no time
    suiting up.
In a mirror, I looked at my fairly flat tummy and thick full head
    of hair,
and wickedly hoped that Jeanny might be sporting a belly and
    toupee ——
I'm bad that way.
I arrived at the restaurant a wee bit early and was given a table
that afforded me an insider's view of the kitchen.
I had bought a French newspaper and pretended to be able to
    read it
while I sipped the vin de maison, waiting for Jean.
I was no tourist and was not about to look it.
I belonged.

Soon there was a commotion at the entrance to the restaurant
and the owner and maitre d' and waiters all ran to greet the patron.
It was yes — of course —— Jean-Jacques.
I had to admit to myself — grudgingly — that he did look good ——
Better than he had in school.
And I mused, "If only I had so many friends who were waiters."
He took notice of me and in his exaggeratedly rugged and
    graceful way
he sashayed over — all the way revealing his grossly overperfect teeth.
Like a demented Osmond.
And then he gave me one of those suspiciously affectionate
    European greetings.
Like a homosexual might.
He commented immediately on my attractive floral shirt and
    Bermuda shorts
and said he had the same make of camera.
"Thank you" — I glibly replied.
He said there was a table for us at the window.
I insisted we stay at my table because I enjoyed the convenience
of being so close to the cutlery station.
He agreed all too readily.
He wants something — I mused again.
We ordered —— Jean ordered.
And we exchanged recapitulations of our lives since our last meeting
and enjoyed some genuinely amusing reminiscenses.
Jean worked in the Canadian Embassy and everything seemed fine.
If there were any crises he wasn't letting on.
He knew how to hurt me.
On and on he went —— we both went.
Soon I was laying my fork and knife at five o'clock, sipping the
    last bit of wine
and still there wasn't even a hint
that there was anything wrong in his life.

My patience broke —— I cleared my throat.

"Look Jean," I said, "I've heard some rumors

that you've gotten yourself into a bit of a bind recently."

"No, no — I've been fine."

"You're sure? No death in the family, no arrest for child
    molestation or anything of that sort?"

"No, no, nothing — where did you hear such a thing?"

"Sources," I rejoined and pressed on, "You're sure you didn't lose
    a lot of money

or that you're not being blackmailed over some photos someone
    may have?"

"No, no — I am nothing like that."

The French will never understand prepositions.

"Everything is wonderful."

I was terror struck.

A crushing wave of sadness came over me.

I had been given misinformation.

A bum steer.

The lunch was over.

He offered to pay for it and after a takeout pie and quiche I'd
    ordered had arrived,

we said our goodbyes and both agreed to do it again — real soon.

Behind his back, I pretended to gag —

I said I was bad.

Back at my hotel, I fell onto my bed — alone — and defeated.

A shaky hand reached for the remote and I turned on the television.

The evenings news had just begun.

To my shock — the lead story was about Jean-Jacques.

Once again the poetic syntax — how do I do it?

Anyway — it seems that Jean had been killed that afternoon

driving his car into a street pole

to avoid hitting an elderly blind woman.

What a hero.

Slowly, the realization that my oldest and dearest friend was dead ——
Overcame me.
The moments that followed are a blur.
I know that I ordered some champagne to calm my frazzled nerves
and during that evening, in every disco and night club I went to,
I noticed for the first time how blind people are to the hurt and
    pain all around them.

On that day, some of the magic went out of Paris for me.
I suppose that's the biggest tragedy of all.

The Guy Next Door

What am I doing up?
Are you kidding?
You can't hear that in there?
Go back to your beauty coma, Mary, 'cause you could use it.
I can't believe you can't hear that.
The Rolling Stones don't make that much noise.
I stand in awe of how the human voice can reach that pitch.
I can hear every moan, every groan, every insertion.
Either those two are wearing body mikes or there's a vagina in
    the next room
with better acoustics than Roy Thomson Hall.
I can't take it anymore.
Every night, every morning.
We're moving.
You be quiet —— I'm talking now.
We have been married for almost 2 years —
    though I'm about 20 years older.
And part of the reason for my accelerated aging process is this place.
I want —— I need something that's our own.
That's mine.
I want to be able to do things without being watched over like a child.
I'm tired of having to borrow things only after someone says,
"Well, as long as you're careful with it, dear."
"Ah, do I have to be? I thought I'd be totally irresponsible with it.
I thought I'd throw it off the roof and take a big crap on it."

Oh, that's terrible.

I am so grateful.

I'm so grateful I can't stand it anymore.

I have to do it all day at work.

"Sir — yes sir, yes, yes, yes, yes."

"Freeman, do you know what I hate more than anything?"

"A yes-man, sir?"

"That's right, Freeman. What do you think of this? It's great, isn't it?"

"Yes sir."

"I like 'ya, Freeman."

And then home — where I should be able to be as undiplomatic
    as I want.

Where I should be able to turd on anything and everything, if I
    so choose.

Oh God, I can't go on with this,

with Hannibal crossing the mountains in there.

Oh no —— here she goes.

It's special, isn't it?

"Oh, it's special — it's special — it's special!"

How can it be special every bloody night of the week?

I don't care if it's your mother and father!

I just don't care anymore.

Obsession

I know what I want to say to her.
I just don't know how to say it
in a way that won't result in her having me arrested.
I just don't think I can play games with her.
It's gone too far in my mind for me to be discreet and subtle.
In there we've already done it hundreds of times
    in every way, shape and form you can imagine
—— And some you wouldn't want to.
Some of them are just that beautifully filthy.
I just know that if I went up to her, that anything
I'd planned to say would evaporate —
all my sweet and sensitive ways
would be savaged by the lustful animal that I really am
and I'd hear myself grunting:
"Woman — woman — for God's sake let's stop this mutual torture
and realize that the only thing that is keeping us apart
is your vicious desire to drive me out of my mind.
So for pity's sake let's do it.
Let's abandon politeness and self-control
and give ourselves over to my every desire.
Let's go at each other till we hemorrhage.
Like lonely mink.
Locked in my bedroom.
Flesh on flesh —
Sweat drenched till we dehydrate —
and are left as nothing but carnally satiated dust."

Oh yeah ——

I'm alright.
I'll be OK.

As an approach it's a little over the head.
I know.
It's too much, too soon.
But I don't know how to go about getting this woman.
I mean, I've always known what to say to other women —
because other women are just — women.
But this person possesses the single finest piece
of female anatomy I've ever known.
And she's keeping it all to herself.
She should share it.
She's selfish.
She should give it to me.

I'm alright.
I'll be OK.

No — I won't.
Not till she and I are one being fused forever.
Which is not going to happen until I figure out a way
to charm her —— to be sensitive — kind — provocative — witty —
    taller —
much better looking than I am ——
Till I figure out a way to become you.
Ah — most of the time I feel perfectly adequate not being you.

But this time — forget the modesty.
When you walk into a room something happens.
Legs cross — there's not a dry seat in the house.
Ardently heterosexual men start doubting it.
Born agains — die again.
And then your approach ——
You breeze up — smile — maybe wink — let them gaze at your
    form —
throw up some wit — let off some flattery.
Then the offer ——
Spot of dinner — a little theatre maybe.
A little drink afterwards and then home to have your babies.
They fall at your feet —— I've seen it.
I have to beg.
Plead.
I use guilt — sympathy.
Yes — "I am dying" — is the best line I have.
The words "malignant tumor" and "open sesame"
serve basically the same function in my sex life.
I can't do that with her though.
I can't kill off my grandmother again.
I can't lie.
It's too real.
It's too much.
I can't go on.
I have to have this woman.
I have to.

I'm alright.
I'll be OK.

Haute Couture

Look, I haven't sold out.
I haven't changed.
It just looks like I have.
It's a lie, but it's a lie I like.
It's a lie that gets me places ——
Like people's bedrooms.
Underneath, however, I'm still the same semi-revolutionary
that you've always known and loved to disagree with.
Still the same man whose personal style used to answer very closely
to the description of the average bag lady.
Whose beard and hair used to make his little cousins call him Jesus.
A man who, by the way, liked that very much.

But I had to grow up and live in the real world —
no matter how corrupt we may think it is.
And, whether you believe it or not —
politically correct and socially inept don't have to be synonymous.
You can think left and dress right.
Dressing badly doesn't help feed the poor.
It just makes you look like them.
Besides, when it comes down to it, there's only one motivation
        for my chic altered state
and that's my rather substantial libido.
My killer concupiscence.
Raw lust.

Something a hyperactive liberal like yourself
should consider a sign of extreme mental health.
What you see on my body are not just designer clothes, but a
    stylish reflection of my desire
to have an incredible amount of sex
with an incredible number of women
who look absolutely incredible.

Let's face it.
The women in our movement aren't — aren't ——
They are nice
They are dedicated.
And they have more hair in their noses than I have on my head.
Sexist?
No.
Perceptive?
Yes.

You see, I grew tired of an appearance
that would turn well-adjusted women into rape-obsessed neurotics
if I went for a walk at night.
I was tired of being directed to the loading door by maitre d's.
And I started to develop a taste for — a need for —
people who look good.
People who expend a lot of energy on — looking good.
They may not always be overly socially conscious.
Sometimes it's hard to tell if they're conscious at all.
But I get tired of thinking all the time.
And with them I don't have to.

You know, I've always had a bent for pretty inanimates — so it's
    only natural
that I should develop a bent for pretty animates as well.
And to get near them — near enough to touch — you have to
    dress well.
It's their gauge of your worth as a human being.
They don't care if you can turn a phrase ——
They want to know where you got your boots.
So their biggest purpose in life is to display clothes.
So they're mannequins.
They're mannequins who put out.
And you can turn your anarchistic nose in the air,
but I freely admit that there is a facet of my personality
that very much enjoys standing, posing, looking good,
and being seen with people who look even better.
I enjoy these women and even the men — now and then —
because they are more than content to sit silently in their lovely
    linens —
attentions riveted to my every witty word.
Speaking only occasionally to giggle out a much appreciated,
"Oh you're so funny."

It's me in my glory.

Video Dating

OK — I guess.
Is it on?
Does it have to be into the camera?
I mean, right into the camera?
Couldn't I pick a spot or something?
I guess — yes.
I prefer that.
OK — anything?
OK — well, I guess a little background ——
I began as a union of an ovum and a sperm and I've made little
    progress since.
I'm just a two-legged slug with a penchant for ludes.
My mother used to say, "It doesn't really do much.
It just sort of sits there and makes a mess."
Well, I guess — who better than our moms to define our lives?
The mess gets more complicated.
It's a cosmopolitan mess now —
but it's still a mess — I guess.

When I was 8 I expressed a great deal of interest and enthusiasm
in becoming a sous chef.
It was the sign of life my parents had been looking for.
Crib death had been conquered — I guess.
All the same, they ended in divorce.

I come from a broken home. Mom's in six pieces, Dad's in eight
and our kitchen and living room are spread from coast to coast.
I have one and a half sisters — one whole one and one half:
just legs, some lips and some hair —
embarrassing as hell to kiss.
I guess I'm just kidding to put you at ease —
to say that I'm well adjusted —
despite my fractured home life as a youth.

I guess I was a fairly normal teenager.
I sweated a lot.
And I smelled quite bad.
And I had a very strange belief no one on earth understood me.
I smell pretty good these days ——
I'm dry and I know two or three people
who have a rough idea of what's going on up here.
I guess I hated my mother — well, I didn't really.
Well — like every good teen.
It's just that she had this way of getting in the way
of my teenaged angst ——
I had lots.
But, as you grow older, and contempt becomes toleration —
    even respect —
you get Christmas without knife throwing and Easter without
    bloodletting ——
It's great.

I've looked for purpose in life once or twice
and a job not nearly so often.

I guess I've always found people to be as silly as party hats
and as pathetic as dogs with no legs.

I ski well, I enjoy movies, and plays, cooking, reading ——
And I have an enormous dick.
And — hell — I guess that's me — I guess.

Can we stop?
I really don't have much more to say.

How long does it usually take?

On The Edge

OK — OK —
Don't anybody move.
I said — don't move.
Don't.
Of course it's a gun.
What am I supposed to have? Twisted pantyhose?
I'm going to strangle you all to death?
Keep the police at bay and then turn them on myself?
What are you — nuts?

Alright now, let's not lose our heads — or we just may — literally ——
Savvy — know what I mean?
So, let's just calm down — take a deep breath —
just for a moment send our thoughts somewhere else —
some place warm and sunny —
with a person in a grass skirt serving us Mai Tais.
Yes, like a beach. Thank you, ma'am.
That's quite an imagination you have.
How about if I say a word and you say the first thing that comes
      to mind —
and we'll play instant association games all bloody afternoon.
What are you, nuts?
I have a gun.
I am a man with a gun.
I am a psycho. What are you, nuts?

You don't yell out beach to a man with a gun.
Use your brain.

OK, ease it down —— calm yourself.
Now, you may be wondering — why we're here.
Why is this person doing this?
What is wrong with our world that leads a man to do this?
Of course you're wondering that.
What are you supposed to be thinking about?
Your shoe size? What am I, nuts?
OK — that was rhetorical. Nobody answer.
I'll answer ——
Of course I'm nuts.
Sane people do this?
Sane people start wars, huh?
No they don't.
I'm turning this into a Greenpeace rally — any Pro-Choicers here?
Let's have a party.
We'll pick up a few anti-nukes, a couple of gays,
and we'll move this baby down to city hall.
What do you say?
I'm going out of my mind ——

Ah jeez — what the hell am I doing?
This is strange.
If you knew me you'd be really surprised.
This is not like me.
I guess I just want some attention.
That's so obvious, I know — but it's that simple.
I just need somebody to say, "Hey, you're alright — you dress nice."
I go to a lot of trouble.

Like my hair...it's a lot of work.
Do — do ya — like this? It's flattering, eh?
Too short?
You again.
You are nuts, lady.
The rest of you can go ——
'Cause we are going one on one, lady.
I have a gun.
My hair is perfect.
I look fucking wonderful.
What are you? In the pay of my mother?
All I wanted was a little attention — a little time.
What did I have?
Nothing.
TV and Lego.
Scooby Doo — Scooby Doo, where are you?
Who cares?
What kind of role model is that for a child?
Four kids in a van.
Where's the morality?
You mind telling me what's in a Scooby Snack?
I'm a loon.
Nothing's going right.
I forgot to wear deodorant today — and I worry so much —
so much that I sweat three times as much as usual.
My zipper's down all the time.
Nothing's the way it's supposed to be.
I'm not finished —— don't move.
I look into the future. I was supposed to get married —
and have a job and a kid — the same color as me —
but I don't see it.

I see me dying friendless in a boarding house —
        smoking rollies with my legs crossed —
in a housecoat, playing gin rummy with a war vet.
That's not a future ——
That's a documentary by an angry, young film student.
Look — I'm sorry.
I've had a rough day.
You know, things build — and you just want
to mow down a crowd and terrorize the people.
Get it off your chest.
I'm imperfect.
I'm nuts.
And so are you.

What a statement.

A Sensitive Man

I did.
I saw it.
It's a beautiful, beautiful thing.
A beautiful baby.
It's very fortunate to have the parents that it does.
And, you know, when I picked it up and held it, so fragile and
     beautiful —
I had one of those revelations
that we sensitive men are known for.
You know — it happens when you see a nice sunset.
Or hold a baby.
Or read Rod McKuen.
It's something a macho man could never understand.
It puts us on a different plane of consciousness.
It's when we have our most profound thoughts.
It's when we make those wonderful omelets that sensitive men
     are known for.

Anyway, I was holding this baby — and it came to me.
I thought ——
Look how it treats these people. It spits at them.
It cries, wakes them up at all hours of the night.
It wallows in its own excrement like we wallow in self-pity.
It brings in what? Thirty bucks a month? —— What's that?
It's not something you talk to.
I mean, you wouldn't bring it your problems.
It's never travelled.

It can't dance ——
Never given a brunch.
The thing is, by all normal standards of intelligence — fairly lacking.
But — it's worshipped.
Those two adore it.
I adore it.
I love it.
They love it.
All it has to do is scream its head off for a matter of seconds
and a human nipple — a female human nipple no less —
is placed in its mouth.
I mean, the kid has something going for it.
But, despite all that, despite all his drawbacks ——
Everyone who sees him loves him.
Every noise he makes is listened to and every need he has is fulfilled.
But, when he's grown up — and he's travelled ——
When he's given brunches — and damned good ones ——
When he knows who he is, and where is is ——
Despite all that —
he'll be very, very lucky to get even a few people to love him.
Very few of his noises will be listened to.
And very few of his needs will ever be fulfilled.

And then — the revelation ended.
And like all sensitive men, my thoughts turned to my penis
and where I would put it next.

You know, I think if it weren't for sunsets and little babies
and, well, Rod McKuen — sensitive men would always have erections
and omelets would never get made.
The best we could do would be toasted westerns.
And what kind of a world would that be?

Peace